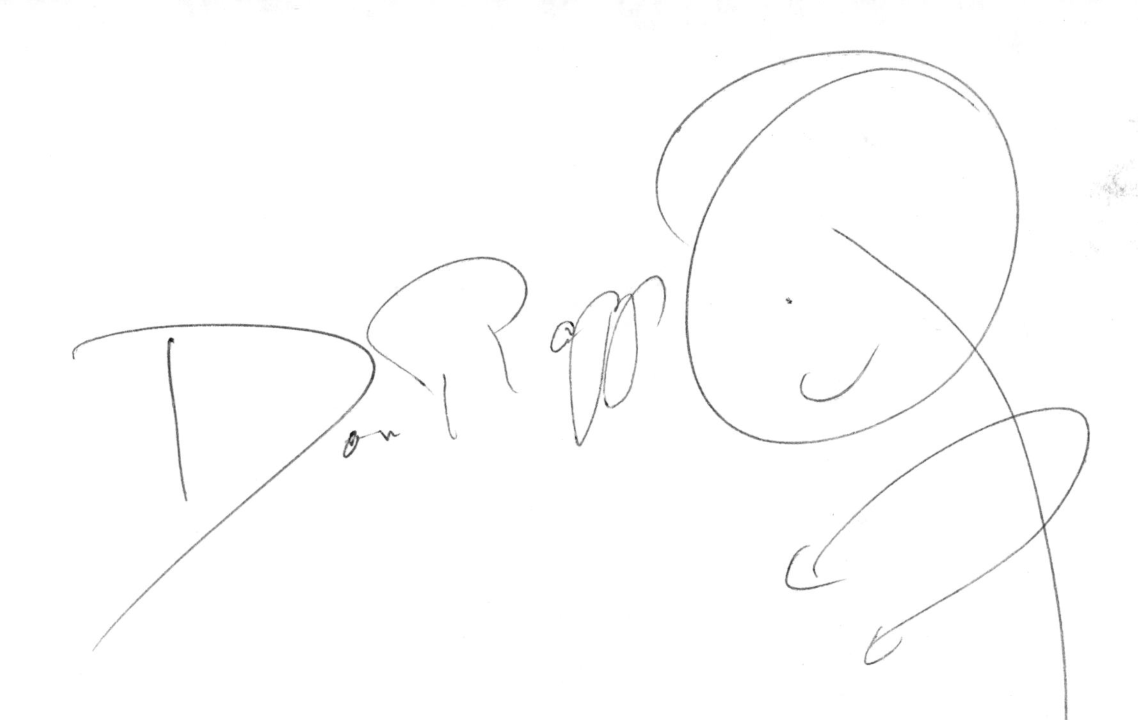

I dedicate this book to those
universally abstract,
yet practical principles
that undergird our planet,
and all us bio-units there on.

Fulcrum Press

Photography - Patsy Rapp
Model - Don Rapp
Cover - Randy Helms

Printed at

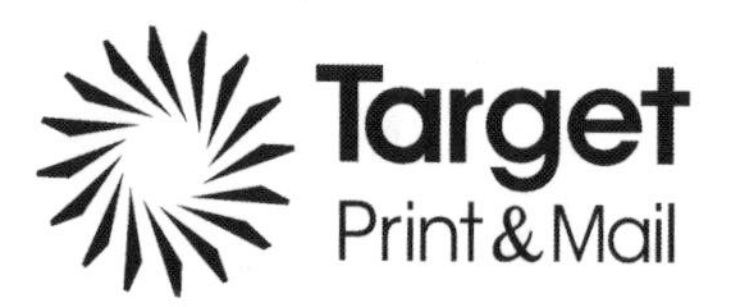

635 West Tennessee Street
Tallahassee, Florida 32304
hello@targetprintmail.com | www.targetprintmail.com

ISBN 978-1-4243-3755-2

This book presents balance exercises and activities that may or may not be right for you. In view of the complex, individual, and specific nature of health and fitness problems, this book is not intended to replace professional medical advice. Every individual is different. **Before starting any exercise program, get your doctor's approval. The publisher** and the author expressly disclaim any responsibility for any loss or risk incurred as a consequence of the application of the contents of this book.

First Printing: March 2007
Second Printing: August 2007
Third Printing: May 2008
Fourth Printing: March 2009
Fifth Printing: March 2010
Sixth Printing: June 2011
Seventh Printing: March 2012
Eight Printing: March 2013
Ninth Printing: May 2014
Tenth Printing: September 2015
Eleventh Printing: May 2016
Twelfth Printing: September 2017

Table of Contents

Acknowledgement of the Core Four

I will try to do justice to these four and to the many more in Appendix A.

Javos Barnett was my American College of Sports Medicine certification teacher. He was an inspirational person, committed to health and most helpful to me, as the oldest one in class. Javos had a delightful personality, an infectious laugh, and willingly shared his tremendous store of health science knowledge.

The second was Bill Serow, a bright and joyful thinker. He gave me a kick in the seat of the pants to complete this book. I am indeed indebted to both Javos and Bill. Both died too young.

It is a joy to thank this third person, Patsy, my wife of over 50 years. How in the heck can any man thank his wife for being so supportive? My being an author was and is hard work for her. I am normally crazy enough, but during the writing process . . . wow! Also, thanks to Patsy for her photo work and her choice of the least expensive model in the world.

Since 1954, I have enjoyed an academic relationship with R. Buckminster Fuller. Actually, to my edification, we talked on several occasions. He inspired me toward thinking creatively, and encouraged life-long motivation to think openly about the wonders of the Universe and all its contents. He wrote the following four lines, which will tell you why I am so indebted to his Universal thoughts.

The environment to each must be
every thing that isn't me.
The universe, in turn must be,
everything that isn't me . . . plus me.
Fuller

All of us are equally endowed with Fuller's "plus me." We are designed to add uniqueness to the Universe. Your *life-long health* is important; your *balance* is crucial, And, indeed, your *very being is* of unique value.

Note: Poems and quotes are the author's unless other authorship is given.

The Spawning Ground of this Book.

When I read a book, I like to know where do the author's ideas come from. Briefly, here I am in one page.

- High School and College basketball and track
- Bachelor's degree in Physical Education
- Army training and duty as a Physical Therapy Specialist
- Masters degree in Early Childhood Education
- First male public school kindergarten teacher in the State of Florida
- Ph.D. in Child Development
- Taught 34 years University Child Development. Gerontology and Creativity
- Year-long Behavior Science Fellowship at Shands Medical Center, Gainesville FL
- An American College of Sports Medicine class for Exercise Leader sparked interest in the neurology of balance
- Juggler since 1940 to date
- Juggling instructor for twenty summers at the Chautauqua Boys and Girls Club
- American College of Sports Medicine certification as an Exercise Leader and Personal Trainer

My interest in health was spawned by extensive involvement in sports, and cinched by the degree in Physical Education. Even before that, my juggling taught me that the nervous system's ability to learn is accomplished when right practice is diligently practiced. All of this education and experience has allowed a fascination with the health of the youth, the elderly, and those with disabilities.

My specific interest in balance was sparked in retirement when I became certified as an exercise leader by the American College of Sports Medicine. The instructor was dynamic, and the content magnificent. The class reinvigorated my interest in anatomy, physiology and kinesiology.

In addition to this, I have been a juggler since 1940. This experience is important in understanding my approach to balance enhancement. I do not teach juggling in balance classes, although you will become aware that the principles of juggling are involved in some activities. But then, human balance is a kind of juggling of our 30 trillion cells, which of course, includes the brain. As you read on you will become increasingly conscious that I encourage the juggling-like skills that underlie coordination competence. Balance, after all, is a motor skill. Competence, with regard to balance, can be enhanced.

Last but far from least, this book is a personal quest for health in general, and specifically, for a lifetime of balance. I, like you, ***do <u>not</u> want to fall***.

Prologue

This book is dedicated to a good life; a life of planning, thinking, doing and sharing. Our nervous system is the basis of our actions. This book is about our nervous system's maintenance and even its enhancement. The good news is that we can be enhanced under almost any but the most stringent of conditions.

I am convinced that the world has yet to comprehend the fabulous nature of our bodies and especially our brains. The brain is one of the most complex, well-designed, efficient, organic, operating systems in the known Universe. However, the magnificence of anything is often taken for granted. I'm also convinced that when we begin to appreciate the potentialities of our bodies and brains we will insist on taking more responsibility for our own optimum health. And yes, we can do a lot to keep ourselves healthy. Our part is to conscientiously facilitate the gifts we have been given.

The book, *The Three Pound Universe,* by Judith Hooper and Dick Teresi likens the human brain to the universe. The comparison is not far-fetched. These authors suggest that the number of possible pathways through the human brain is greater than the number of particles in the Universe. The comparison is not far fetched. Our brain is truly magnificent. The more connected pathways there are in our brain, the better we learn, perform, perceive, and secure our memories. Obviously, our potential is far greater than our present reality.

As we progress in our personal betterment, the ride gets smoother, our vitality is enhanced, and we step toward our health ideal. My desire is to assist you to reach for and acquire better health and balance.

This book will highlight the powerhouse within you. Certainly, we can agree that the longer you live the more good you can do. You can have more health, more balance, and more life. A quality life permits honest pride.

I have taught balance classes since 1999. That is when I coined the term Kinetic Arts Training (KAT). Kinetic means movement. Graceful, safe movement is a dynamic art generated by basic health and frequent motor practice. KAT was purposefully given a broad meaning; i.e., any series of motor skilled movements the mastery of which requires repeated practice. In the process of motor mastery, the brain forms new pathways that render the skilled movements progressively more efficient and consistent.

Introduction

The chapter on Fitness offers reasons for being fit. The Motivation chapter gives hints for staying healthy. The Brain chapter offers facts on the magnificent nature of the brain. And the Balance Control Systems chapter puts forth an understanding of the neurological systems that control balance.

The Knowledge chapter lays out ideas and principles needed for a quality mental and physical life. The Physical Tools chapter details down-to-earth, useable tools you can apply to any immediate or future balance problem.

This book is a very special effort for two reasons. 1. Each and every reader is a special member of my balance class. 2. The content in *On Balance* is my personal quest for health in general, and specifically, for a lifetime of balance. No one wants to fall. This book can help to make our balance better. We are all like Olympic athletes involved in the sport of life. And we are on the first team . . . for life.

On Balance is about creating an ever-better brain, properly bonded to every portion of the body. Kinetic Arts Training (KAT) encourages every nerve in the body to do its best for our balance. When this is done well, the brain moves from a cluttered, tangled jungle of nerve cells toward a highly interrelated network of efficient communicative links. The whole of the body can work together for continuing good balance. If or when you stumble, you want to recover quickly and firmly.

It is not only the presence of the higher brain centers that makes humans different from all other animals, but also the vast number of interconnections that are present and can be generated with learning that gives us our fabulous potential. Persistent practice, *at any age*, can initiate new brain neural connections.

First and foremost, this book is about you, with the emphasis on *all of you.* Balance is the book's topic; you are the subject, and your healthy future is the goal. Its information, exercises, and activities will guide you toward learning new motor skills in the pursuit of better balance.

Falling has a high cost in pain, misery, and money not only for the injured but also for caregivers and society. The purpose of this book is to help you keep your balance and thus reduce the devastation caused by falls.

If you have fallen, you know full well you don't want to do that again. Recovery from a fall takes far too long. Prevention is far cheaper and allows us the magnificent benefits of longer lasting independent mobility. By the same token, if you have never fallen and don't intend to, your efforts to prevent falls are well placed. The goal of KAT is high-level neurological functioning as long as possible. Does not that sound like the famous motto, "Be All That You Can Be?" But, let's make it personal. Reading this book tells me that you are on your way to becoming ***all that you can be***.

Physiologists tell us that at the tender age of 30 years, the nervous system is beginning to lose some of its abilities. However, when we challenge ourselves with some reasonable physical fitness practices, we lose very little until very late in life. Observe some 100-year-olds still playing their musical instruments much as they did in their youth. Practice may not make perfect, but it sure does keep us functioning.

And that is the point of Kinetic Arts Training. KAT is a range of methods, practices and attitudes that lets *you* keep what you have, get back what you had, and remain gloriously independent as long as possible. And there is more, as you will see. The fact you're reading this book shows your intent to do something significant about your own balance and well-being. That intent can positively affect your future.

Kinetic Arts (KA) is an umbrella term covering all biological movement. More specifically, Kinetic Arts Training (KAT) is defined as those exercises, activities, attitudes, and motivations specifically required for physical balance.

KAT is based on neurological realities, exercise mechanics, and a positive philosophy. Balance can be enhanced regardless of age. KAT works with all parts of the nervous system. If one balance system is damaged, KAT works to improve those elements that remain functional. We have the power to delay our age-related declines . . . by a lot.
Before we go any further, let me say that balance is not all in your feet and legs. And it's not just a meticulous avoiding of pitfalls. Poetically, balance is leaping over life's pitfalls fueled by the dance of the soul. Let me explain.

Well-grounded physical balance is controlled by every part of the body, especially your brain. Also, balance is influenced by your attitude, your knowledge, and your motivation to remain independent. When your life is functioning well, you are much more likely to be solid on your feet. If you are ill, depressed, injured and/or in lousy shape, your balance suffers. Failing to enhance the nervous system is also a limiting factor for health. But there is hope. Much can be done to slay the dragon of limitation. This book is about health and especially about the human nervous system that can be made better.

We are all competing with time and gravity and our own attitudes toward improving or at least retaining our quality of life. Athletes become more diligent as their competition nears. The same principle applies to older adults who need to improve their balance. As we progress in age, we must adhere more stringently to correct biological practices. We can retain our biological qualities and even enhance them. Our lifelong Olympic event is a balanced life in all its breadth. In this regard, *growing older is an Olympic sport.* Active and ardent participation is the goal. Said another way:

Falls are inevitable unless balance is the goal.
A balanced life is the goal of the soul.

Independent mobility is a powerful theme. The concept of balance applies to everything from the United States Constitution to teenage maturation. I will share many ways to purposefully move your body with the get-up-and-go of the Energizer Bunny.

What more can I say, I want you around
I want you tomorrow fit, healthy and sound.
You're very important, you are a joy.
So take care of yourself, you're much more than a toy.

Note: You have noticed from time to time I lapse into rhyme. It's not Shakespeare, of course. My intent is to use novelty and rhyme to open the highways of awareness. The above four lines are a small part of a poem about stress. See appendix I for the entire Up Tight poem.

My motivation for writing this book is the same as yours. I don't want to fall. Like you, I want to live with a quality body and mind that controls and experiences movement, thought, and relationships as long as possible. The word *fitness* is an Exercise Science term for high-level physiological order. The word 'order' is a synonym for balance.

Balance and Six Aspects of Human Life

The human entity may be subdivided into six categories: physical, mental, social, emotional, moral and spiritual. Below is a brief explanation of each as they apply to balance. These six are not mutually exclusive. When you positively influence one, all others are influenced. Balance is usually thought of as physical balance alone. However, the word balance has many connotations.

Physical balance refers to the body systems that control our balance. Total physical health is a large part of optimum physical balance.

Mental balance refers to those mental mind-brain processes that keep us on an even keel. To remain buoyantly alive we must face our problems, stay alert to challenges, and judiciously adjust to loss.

Social balance includes trust, deference, tolerance, and empathy. Social balance allows us to think solidly in the heat of disagreements. A balanced body works toward societal cohesion and stability.

Emotional balance allows an accurate comprehension and control of our own feelings, while avoiding pathological and codependent victimhood.

Moral balance includes being cognizant of the rights of others as well as one's own rights within the framework of cultural precedent. Moral balance insists on personal responsibility for our own decisions, behaviors, goals and adjustments.

Spiritual balance takes into account all the afore mentioned before settling on a belief system that is amenable to mature reason. A healthy belief system honors our earthy biology and at the same time offers humble reverence to realities beyond our awareness.

I have taught balance classes since 1999 at Senior Centers, Gyms, and Retirement Villages and have given numerous speeches at a variety of venues. My groups have been extremely varied. Athletes come to my class because they want better balance. Patients with Parkinson's disease appear in class because they are anxious about loss of motor control. Persons with brain injuries, and stroke show up because they desire a brain that functions better. Older persons, as well those in middle age attend class because they want to continue functioning at a high level. Anyone with a reasonably functioning nervous system is a prime candidate for the ideas and activities of Kinetic Arts Training.

This book is merely an idea-link between you and me. We are both on the same path, where joy accumulates as we learn the tricks and skills of balance. Physiologists report that two-legged locomotion is a 'miracle'. With practice, our own efforts reinforce the facility to function better and longer.

KAT can greatly enhance the quality of your life. What a promise, and what a responsibility! I intend to offer good advice, planning, motivation, tools, solid reasoning, and good humor in the journey toward better balance.

Balance requires continual attention to the task. The goal of KAT is to make balance better, or at least to maintain balance as we grow older. It is just plain fun to learn new ways of moving, doing, and standing safe and tall. Going places is your badge of success.

I love the Olympian analogy. It is not just poetic drivel. We are all Olympians in the sport of life. Realistically, advancing age diminishes all our functions. But now we undeniably know that eating better and exercising will slow the aging process. In fact, exercise can make you physiologically younger, with the goal of retaining independent mobility for as long as possible. And that is a goal well worth any effort.

Secure balance is vital to our mobility as two-legged creatures. But balance becomes more difficult with age. This book concentrates on the many ways you can become an Olympian on the court of life. Reading further is the first step in your balance training.

"We are not what we used to be," an older lady told me. Then she spryly added, *"But I'm not dead yet!"* This book is about your *yet*. You have the rest of your life to get better and better. Now we get on with the specifics. Welcome. Jackie Gleason would say it with flair:

"And away we go."

Fitness: What Is It?

For age is opportunity no less than youth itself
though in another dress.
And as the evening twilight fades away
the sky is filled with stars, invisible by day.
From Henry Wadsworth Longfellow's *Morituri Salutamus*

Note: A young Longfellow would never have written this. Henry's sentiment comes clothed in day or evening dress.

Each new day opens new possibilities.
Opportunities come in a variety of dress.

We know that life becomes more difficult as the body ages. Nervous system functions slow down and are more subject to injury and disease. One of the most prevalent causes of this speedy decline occurs because of a new disease recently named, sedentary disease. All of us know someone who is a bona fide couch potato. If it is you, this book can help you shed that reality.

Happily, the speed of neurological decline need not be so fast. Let's say that for some wonderful reason a typical inactive person becomes progressively more active. Often this is because of some emergency. Or perhaps they have caught fire with the awareness that they can become more fit and thus increase their quality of life. We know that when sedentary people become active, they are progressively more productive. They are more physiologically able, more mentally alert, and more emotionally solid. To others they look better, their eye bags recede, and their color is vivid and healthy because their hearts work better. They are pumping more oxygen through their bodies, eliminating better, sleeping better, thinking more positively, and they exhibit all this with positive talk and improved social relations. The immune system has also become more active. General activity is a basic need of the human body.

At birth, we are thrust into the Olympic sport of life. We are on the field for the entire game. There is no second team, no bench, and for our own good, we had better become our own coach. Life is unequivocally a very serious game. You are a winner every time you affirm, *it's time for me to play ball.*

Balance, Aging, Fitness and Lifestyle Choices

Balance demands constant attention; however, our ability to pay attention also diminishes with time. All Kinetic Art Training (KAT) exercises help to maintain our attention skills, which in turn aid in the prevention of falls.

According to an article in the November 1999 *Scientific American, "Muscular Again: Your New Body,"* muscle strength wanes over time, contributing to the likelihood of falling. But muscles can be kept more active, vibrant and strong by using them. The article continues,

"Geriatric health specialists now also see muscle loss as underlying many of the injuries to elderly people caused by falling. Thrown off balance, an older person may not have the muscle power necessary to correct posture quickly enough to avoid a nasty fall."

A partial list of the bad side of falls begins with time spent trying to heal an injury that could have been avoided. Injuries affect us physically, emotionally, socially, and mentally. In all of these areas, loss of function is pervasive and painful. Persons who have been injured have increased anxiety, which may be heaped on loved ones. A fall can cost a great deal in money, pain and loss of independence. Avoiding these negatives is common sense. Being fit means that the heart can handle vigorous exercise. A good heart is the foundation of strong, flexible muscles, and then more controlled balance follows. General fitness is the keystone of a good life. Good health is the lubricant that makes life flow from the word go. I will approach this topic from a variety of angles, but right now, let's start with something provocative.

A philosopher once told me, "During the first half of our lives we are controlled by others, we wrestle with our demons, and we think we're immortal. In the second half of our lives, when and if we overcome these three obstacles . . . all we do is . . . *laugh.*

Laughter is an important component of fitness. I want to laugh a lot, and we are much more likely to laugh when fitness is our intimate companion.

There are many sources for health information today. Yet we are becoming less fit, which is frustrating to say the least. TV shows and popular magazines describe the dangers of smoking and aggressively advertised fad diets, while at the same time they sell fat and sugar . . . *to* children. Paradoxically, most newspapers now print health-related articles. The Sunday *Parade* magazine, for example, carried by many newspapers, regularly runs a series of health related articles by Isadore Rosenfeld M.D. Recently he wrote about diabetes, which has become an epidemic in the United States and a major cause of death. In the last 44 years, the incidence of Type II diabetes (adult onset diabetes) has increased from 1.6 million to 11 million cases, a jump of 700 percent. Children in great numbers are now being diagnosed with Type II diabetes. The cost to all of us is horrendous.

One major cause of diabetes is obesity. Sixty-five percent of Americans are overweight or obese. This group and many others are far from fit and fully healthy. The "baby boomers" will break the bank in health costs if we all don't change for the better. We are experiencing an epidemic of major proportions, one that will affect everyone. Adding insult to injury is an obesity epidemic in children. The good news is that we know that obesity, as well as high blood pressure, may be eliminated or significantly ameliorated by diet control and exercise. An ounce of inexpensive prevention is worth a pound of costly cure.

Proper drug use is part of fitness. For instance, American children consume 80 % of the world's supply of Ritalin, a drug used to treat the symptoms of Attention Deficit Hyperactivity Disorder (ADHD). Daily fatigue from honest exertion, followed by a good night's sleep, can reduce the need for the over prescribed use of drugs like Ritalin.

The larger fitness picture is demonstrated in a statement I heard as an undergraduate, in the 1940s. One of my physical education professors was a runner and health enthusiast. He believed in fitness for life. He told us that a person in good physical condition had a 75 % better chance of surviving an operation than a person in poor physical condition. As a college kid, that statement was informative and inspiring. Today, at my age, it means even more.

My recent certification as an exercise leader and physical trainer by the American College of Sports Medicine prompted my attendance at their annual meeting in Orlando, Florida. Again and again, the research physiologists and physicians at this conference verified my old professor's understanding of the health value to fitness. Who says physical education is a frill?

Exercise experts state that there are four mainstays of wellness.

1. Endurance - Aerobics for the heart health
2. Strength - Resistance training for the muscle strength
3. Flexibility - Stretching for joint range of motion
4. Balance - Challenging, balance oriented stimulation of the entire nervous system along with training for endurance, strength, and flexibility

The first three of the above are largely muscle-oriented. This is good, for they form the basis of good health and balance. However, KAT-like exercises focus directly on the nervous systems, which control balance. KAT is the only one of the four that takes its lead directly from Neurology.

Physiologists are of one mind when they say that exercise is the best place to spend your health dollar.

When asked which is more important, diet change or exercise,
physiologists choose exercise, but add that if you exercise and improve your diet,
you become fit faster.

Research shows that more than 50 % of all disease can be traced to lifestyle choices. (Some say that this figure is as high as 75%.) These estimates prompt the question, what is a lifestyle choice?

Lifestyle choices include decisions about food choices, activity level, and your attitude about life and yourself. For example, wearing a seat belt is a life-saving choice. The opposite is couch potato-ing yourself into loss of muscle and a higher susceptibility to illness.

One recent physiology study particularly impressed me. It tested the oxygen uptake of obese people. The subjects' ability to use oxygen was measured at the beginning of an exercise program, and then again each week. After only one week of moderate exercise, these obviously unfit obese folks increased their ability to use oxygen. Wonder of wonders, the human body quickly and positively adjusts to appropriate lifestyle adjustments.

Even a top athlete's nervous system deteriorates with age. However, the nervous system deteriorates much more quickly in older people who are sedentary. Susan Bovre's excellent book, *Balance Training: A Program for Improving Balance in Older Adults,* echoes this thought. She states:

> "Exercise will not correct all of the changes that have led to impaired balance. Natural aging, chronic conditions, acute illness, or injury all may contribute to decline. Exercise can address ways to prevent falls through improved posture, increased muscle strength, increased motor skills, improved agility, coordination, and improved self-confidence. These components form the basis for balance training."

I would add several points to Bovre's list of contributors to decline. They are bad habits, sedentary life style (disuse), poor health decisions, limited range of joint motion, and unforgiving environments. I 've tried to find a more encouraging way to say it but we do deteriorate, *Biology makes its own rules.* The good news is that we can do much to overcome age-related decline. According to Bovre, "Fifty percent of the decline that has been attributed to aging is actually due to the disuse that is labeled secondary aging. Abuse, as in smoking, sun overexposure, alcohol, drugs, and overeating, also results in intensified aging."

Exercise, the physiologists tell us, is the best way to lose weight. *Weight* rhymes with "give it the *gate.*" *Health* rhymes with *wealth.* Read the following and see what I mean:

Plan to stay healthy. Say good-bye to your fat.
Slim, trim, fit and slender, now that's just where it's at.

Note: I admit my "poetry" is often "cutesy." But please consider its serious intent.

The Tufts Center for Aging has listed 10 "markers" for aging. They are:

Aerobic capacity
Blood sugar tolerance
Blood pressure
Body temperature regulation
Body-fat percentage
Bone density
Strength
Basal Metabolic Rate (BMR)
Lean Body Mass
Total HDL & Cholesterol level.

Physicians, exercise scientists, physiologists and cardiac surgeons agree with the Tufts Center that all 10 markers can be improved with exercise. I love this list, but they left out *balance.* Yes, even balance requires a healthy foundation in overall fitness. Many younger non-exercisers don't know the value of exercise either. If they knew and understood this list, exercise would become a lifelong habit.

Now let's become a little more specific and approach motor fitness directly. We all have had pivotal events in our lives. I enrolled in an American College of Sports Medicine physiology and strength training class. The class material contained a five-word definition of motor fitness: *agility, balance, coordination, power* and *speed.* All five are interrelated and complementary.

Lack of any one of these abilities is a marker of the aging process. All five must remain viable to keep the body and mind alert, strong, flexible, and durable. Together they promote long-lasting balance, which is demonstrated by more accurate and fluid locomotion.

For memorization purposes, how about the acronym A B C P S, *agility, balance, coordination, power* and *speed.* Later, I shall give more detail on each and how their memorization can help you become more fit and balanced.

On the surface, some KAT exercises seem to have little to do with the complexities of balance. (See the chapter on Physical Tools). However, upon deeper examination, one realizes that the intent of these exercises is to improve the functioning of the whole nervous system. When any part of the nervous system is improved, there is a concomitant improvement in overall functioning. The trick is to prescribe and perform exercises that are the most relevant to each person's particular need. But when you practice alone, you become your own trainer. This means that you work on what you cannot do. The work out plan needs to proceed in small steps with frequent practice.

The qualities of health and fitness are very much associated. *The 30-Minute Fitness Solution*, by Joann Manson and Patricia Amend, tells us some astounding facts. Regular moderate physical activity at least 30 minutes a day reduces:

risk of premature death by 30 to 50%
heart disease by 30 to 50%
osteoporosis (in women) by 40 to 50%
stroke by 30% - 50%
type two diabetes by 30% - 40%
colon cancer (in women) by 20% - 30%
breast cancer by 30% - 50%

Taking to heart these figures will increase your motivation to follow a healthy path. The KAT goal of all exercise is neurological rejuvenation and integration. Thus, all challenging exercises lay a foundation for good balance.

There is no pill that will do as much good as exercise. In fact, when sedentary people begin a program, they can often reduce or eliminate some of their drug dependencies. Exercise offers multiple payoffs. Sweat is good for more than cleansing your pores.

The Six Aspects of Human Life

The introduction briefly described the *physical, mental, emotional, social, moral* and *spiritual* components of our being. These dimensions are so important to health that they deserve a more detailed examination.

The field of Child Development has long suggested the importance of these six aspects of human complexity. The six are not mutually exclusive. When any one of these six components is improved, all the others benefit. They influence each other, unifying our mind and body. However, for the sake of balance, it is good to work on each one separately, then in combination. These categories are so ingrained in human culture that most cultures have created respectable and useful niches for each. For example, a strongly socially minded person may be an excellent salesperson, or a strong mental person may become a mathematician or philosopher. But the physical is the basis of all the other five. Although one may be dominant, full health is attained when all six are in reasonable balance. It is obvious that the word *balance* has many connotations.

Physical balance consists of the upright, two-legged stance. It deals with the body systems that control balance. But it must be emphasized that overall physical health and fitness is a must for optimum balance. Occupations associated with the physical are physicians, physical therapists, massage therapists, occupational therapist, and physical trainers.

Mental balance consists of harmonious and productive thinking. It includes the brain processes and thought patterns that keep us on an even keel. To remain afloat in life, we must balance innumerable decisions and make millions of adjustments. When problems confront people who are mentally balanced, they boldly face them. Occupations dealing with this aspect of balance include psychiatrists, brain surgeons and researchers, mathematicians, teachers, or tutors.

Emotional balance includes sound and reasonable reactions to disquieting feelings. An emotionally balanced person accurately comprehends and controls emotions, while avoiding actions leading to pathological, and codependent behavior. Occupations relating to emotional balance include psychotherapists, motivational speakers, and grandmothers as good listeners.

Social balance is necessary for cooperative and empathetic relationships. This aspect of balance promotes trust, deference, tolerance, and empathy. A balanced society is one with cohesion and stability. Social balance allows us to think solidly in the face of heated differences of opinion. Socially oriented occupations include ballroom dance instructors, marriage and relationship counselors, and school counselors.

Moral balance permits awareness of and a civil response to cultural norms as well as extremes, such as fads. Morality is a requirement for being cognizant of other's rights as well as your own rights within the framework of cultural precedent. Moral balance involves personal responsibility for your own decisions, behaviors, goals and adjustments. Occupations dealing with this aspect of balance may include, ethics professors, advice columnists, wise parents and friends, Scout leaders, police, and counselors and ministers of all faiths. There is the essence of morality in the very intimate 'still small voice' that hopefully is loud enough to be heard.

Spiritual balance allows us to benefit from support from beyond our full awareness. It enriches, broadens and brings focus to what too often appears as corrosive chaos. Our body is a dynamic bio-temple to be cared for in every way possible. Occupations in this realm would be theologians, professors of religion, and holy men and women of all faiths.

Note: Geithner's, January 2007 excellent article in the American College of Sports Medicine Journal: *Personal Balance: Its Importance and How to Achieve It*, `supports and extends the balance concept as here promoted.

Please keep in mind all five aspects as we consider physical balance. All will help you create your own ways to integrate your intentions, your planning, and your practice. Any loss of physical function is discouraging. But the fact that we can choose to do something about it is a basis for hope. Deep understanding generates stability in all six categories, and helps us realize they are all interrelated and work best when unity of body and mind are promoted.

A Presbyterian minister, Dr. Lloyd Rediger, in his book, *Fit To Be a Pastor* echoes this point. He strongly suggests that a sound religious message is optimized by persons who obviously have balanced all aspects of their being. No one who has significantly neglected one or more of the six facets of life can be a healthy, well-rounded, human spiritual model. What is true for ministers is true for us. We are all ministers of our own health and life.

Again, when the six aspects of balance are unified in health, the road to success is very straight indeed. When all body systems work in harmony with each other, their interconnection becomes stronger. The outcome is seen as grace, tranquility and integrity.

Here is an example of body unity from scientific research. A researcher asked an older group of men to lift weights with one leg but not the other. The exercises were designed to strengthen the quadriceps (the front upper thigh muscle). The weight-lifting leg grew in size and strength. But the non-exercised leg also grew in size and strength (although not as much as the exercised leg). The point is that the body comprises a true unity of functions, all working for the whole and for the life of the individual. When any one of the many systems of the body is made better, all the other systems benefit by their designed interconnection.

The unity of the body should not seem strange. We know that the whole of the universe is interconnected by light and gravity. The body mirrors this miraculous interlacing. But instead of using light and gravity, the body connects its parts with nerves, chemicals, structures, thoughts, and probably forces not yet understood. The human body, like the universe, is characterized by its complexities.

Waneen Spirduso, EdD, of the University of Texas reports a study showing that people under 50 years of age notice very little neurological loss. But, as we reach our 60's and 70's, our yearly decline increases. Spirduso reminds us that by keeping in good neuromuscular condition we can cut that decline in half, which requires a life style decision. Her classic textbook is *Physical Dimension of Aging.*

Chronological age is not the only factor in declining function. The phrase *use it or lose it* comes up again and again in even the most sophisticated books and research papers. A most interesting research compared above average fit 70-years-olds with below average 40-years-olds. The two groups were compared on many physiological measures. The older group was found to be more fit and healthy than the younger group. Good physiological fitness is the basis of a resounding quality of life. Life is not over till it's over. That's a fitness fact.

We begin to lose muscle strength at age 30. By the age of 70, the average person is half as strong as at 30. Notice the word *average*. We can choose to be better than our age-related average. Yes, we lose neurological functioning, muscle mass and reaction speed because of disease, injury, non-use and advancing age. We can, however, control what we choose to do and/or refuse to do. Again, life style choice makes a huge difference.

Witness those circus performers, entertainers, and musicians who are still performing phenomenal physical and mental feats of dexterity well into their 70s and beyond.

Let me remind you of, the tightrope artist Karl Wallenda, the comedian George Burns, the violinist Itzhak Perlman, the artist Grandma Moses, and many others. Super-healthy people can be found in every community. Many older people keep their abilities viable by using them and not abusing them. These exceptional people have used it and they still have it, well into their old age. Practice may not make perfect, but it sure does keep us functioning.

Playful exercise will keep you on the playground longer,
and that can mean a lot of fun.

Frequency - Intensity – Duration (F I D)

The FID prescription is an easy way to remember how to safely plan your exercise.

Frequency = *how* often *you practice.*
Intensity = *how* hard *you practice.*
Duration. = *how* long *you practice.*

The *Use It or Lose It* principal is embodied in FID. A good coach never allows athletes to practice in an unsafe manner. When you are your own balance coach, you are responsible for the frequency of your practices, as well as their intensity and duration. All three control the safety of your exercise. The KAT motto is inherent in FID: *Do what you can, and then a little bit more.*

The nervous system is very different in structure and function from muscles, but both muscles and nerves respond positively when rightly challenged. That challenge is abbreviated with the phrase, *use-it-or–lose-it.*

Let's make FID practical. An example of frequency might be walking twice a day rather than once. When walking more often becomes comfortable, experiment with intensity by walking more vigorously, walking faster, walking up hills, and so forth. Then try walking a bit longer, which is duration. Instead of taking just one turn around the block, walk a little farther each day each time you walk. You can do a lot when patience, persistence and practice are blended.

This down-home story shows how FID works with the principle of growth. A sixteen-year-old farm boy was given a calf to raise. On the first day of its life, he put the calf on his shoulders and lifted it. The next day he did the same thing. As the days passed, the calf gained a lot of weight. It soon was heavier than the boy, but he continued his bovine weight lifting and you know the outcome. The boy got stronger as the calf grew larger. Incremental challenges lead to mental and physical growth. The story never tells just how much the cow weighed when he could not lift it any longer, because that's not the point. The point is, *do what you can, then a little bit more.* All the boy had to do was stay with the project. Our human container responds nicely to gradually increasing challenges.

KAT tools perform the same function as the calf did, but instead of muscles, they concentrate on making the nervous system more responsive. There are many KAT tools, such as balls, batons, cones, lines on sidewalks, etc. (See the chapter: Kinetic Arts Training Tools and Suggested Usage.) Your job is to try to work with some or all of the KAT equipment, and do what you can, at least a couple of times during each exercise session, which is *frequency.* Then come back to it later, with more determination, and try it with greater *intensity.* When you have gained even a small bit of proficiency, work toward greater *duration.* It takes time and repetitive practice to generate the new brain patterns that allow you to perform a skill smoothly and efficiently.

Those who regularly train their bodies in flexibility, aerobics, strength and balance, and who follow a reasonable diet will discover above-average fitness outcomes. Today, more people than ever are walking, enjoying resistance training, and staying with a responsible diet. These people will experience fewer falls and less disease, and their quality of life will be decidedly better and for longer. The idea of exercise even turns up when planning vacations. Tourist agencies tout the health benefits of taking walking tours of the Cotswolds, Tuscany, or the Swiss Alps. Have you ever walked through a large museum? Now that's exercise. I would suggest taking a walk around your local mall or your block before you tackle the exertion of a worthwhile vacation.

Metabolism and Resistance

An informative way to approach fitness is to think of your metabolism. *Metabolism* is defined as the body's ongoing chemical interactions that provide the needed energy to sustain life. *Resting metabolism* is that portion of the overall energy usage required for only the basic needs of the body at rest. *Low metabolism* means you use very few calories to keep your basic function going. Resistance training builds muscle mass.

Muscles require more calories (energy) than fat. When muscle mass is raised and fat is lowered, you burn more calories per minute all day and night. Optimum metabolism allows more strength, and more endurance, to cope with urgent situation.

Metabolic rate increase is not the only answer to losing weight and staying trim. Another is body composition. When your ratio of fat to muscles is right for you, you feel better and you don't have to balance all that excess flab. Weight lifting, walking, water aerobics, or being extra-diligent in your garden or volunteer work all require energy and thus consume calories. Here are some figures. One pound of fat contains 3500 calories. Eating just 100 fewer calories each day and exercising just enough to consume 100 calories more each day will reduce your weight by about two pounds a month. Think about calorie loss process this way: *if it is to be, it is up to me.* Yes, you are your own boss.

Here is a story of hope. An overweight woman told me she went to her doctor, not for a diet, but for a healthy supply of patience. Her doctor understood. She received authoritative support, which gave her the shot of self-confidence she needed to change her lifestyle. He gave her a calorie chart and an exercise pep talk, which was the ammunition she needed to ditch her sedentary way of life. A year later, she returned clothed in the dress size she rightly deserved.

That shot of patience did it. Her motivation was her Doctor's note he had given her.

"Frame this, hang it up, and read it often."

"Take it slow. You did not put on your fat in a minute
and it will not come off in a minute. Increase your
daily exercise a little and reduce your calories a little.
Go especially light on the saturated fats.
You have the rest of your life to get better."

And he signed it legibly and with "**you can do it**". My comment: Now that's an enlightened physician.

She was firmer, looked better, and felt 10 years younger. The next time she came to see her doctor, he gave her a big hug. (Weight losers always give and get hugs.) How did she do it? She knew a lot to start with. She knew that the human body requires a well-rounded daily supply of proteins, carbohydrates, fats, fiber, minerals, water and, oh yes, exercise. Her doctor had told her:

> "Don't call it a diet, rather call it a common-sense investment in health. A strict diet is like a sledgehammer. You don't need a hammer, all you need is time and the persistence that I know you have. Go for it."

Before she left the office, he handed her another poem. She read it later and often on her road to recovery.

Fat accumulates on my hips.
Awful and ugly those cellulite blips.
I've tried to lose 'em but I just can't.
The fatter I get the more I pant.

A friend said you need to get started.
But I'm flabby, I said, I'm even weak hearted.
I get up from the couch and soon need a nap.
I know what you're thinking, I 'm just a fat sap.

I know I should change, I vow to do better.
I want to be lively, a real go-getter.
I'll join the gym and lose some weight.
My goal is health before it's too late.

But first there's lots of work to do.
Then soon my body will be brand new.
So please be there with active support.
My eventual reward? A fancy resort.

Some Nutrition Hints

The latest government food pyramid is right up to date with the best health research. For the first time they have placed exercise at the base of the pyramid. Both vigorous exercise and correct dietary intake are a dynamic duo for health.

Recently I attended a dietary conference at The Florida State University Department of Nutrition and Exercise Science. Every speaker emphasized that exercise and nutrition are the two legs of health. The latest research confirms that counting calories is a simple way to lose weight, but is only part of the solution. A healthy body comes faster if you add some exercise. Diet and exercise are a winning team. A good hint is to avoid those super-sized servings. It's okay to doggy-bag half of it.

We generally don't perceive water and oxygen as filling nutritional needs. But they are both essential to health. Water and oxygen have similar qualities. Both are necessary for us to function well. They lubricate, support, energize, and dispose of wastes. Most of us don't get enough of either. Bob Greene, a much-in-demand physical trainer, states that 80 % of us aren't drinking enough water. Lack of oxygen causes weakness, and when this lack is prolonged, the brain is severely damaged. The Rx is: *Drink water and breathe, and you will feel relieved.* The best things in life are free, and water and air are readily available

There are many sources for health information. A speech by Banana George Blair was inspirational. Banana George Blair is an 85-year-old professional bare-foot water skier at Cypress Gardens, Florida. Below are his five W's for health improvement:

1. ***Water*** – Dehydration: inadequate water supply. For health's sake, drink water.
2. ***Waste*** – Constipation diminishes your zest and brings on grouchiness. Fiber it out!
3. ***Weight*** – Being overweight or underweight generates many negatives. It takes time to get it right. Keep at it.
4 & 5. ***Whole Wheat*** – Whole grains are good. Natural fiber is tasty, even without sugar.

(Whole Wheat is counted as two W's. The broad meaning of four and five is to eat all grains, not just wheat.)

> Note: The name Banana stems from his fancy banana yellow cowboy boots, bandana, and hat. He gives away bananas, which are, by the way, very healthy.

His four W's make his health point; however, I will take the liberty to add four additional W's. First is the factor of Wow. Wow is enthusiasm, a life long youthful exuberance toward life, love, and learning. Two is Wonder, which is more pensive, contemplative, and kind of gentle but relentless quest for more knowledge and understanding of our place in the universe. Three asks, Why are things the way they are, and just where and when, and how can I make them better? And four energizes Willingness to perform the other eight with verve and fortitude.

Perhaps only Wow and Wonder needs more explanation. One reason that children learn more per minute than adults is their inherent Wow of Wonder. Retaining our child-like wonder is good for health, plus it is the yellow brick road to becoming wonderful.

A large amount of health information appears in the popular press. Too often, the full 'truth' is lost in the translation from academic research to the popular press. Have patience with what is said to be a breakthrough. Know that the human body is so complex that all suggestions aren't for everyone. But for your health's sake, think about all possibilities with yourself in mind.

Begin a Fitness Program with Patience and Persistence

Here's a piece of general advice to exercise beginners. Be gentle in your approach. You did not get out of shape in a minute and you cannot get back in shape in a minute. Patience is a virtue, as we learned from the calf-lifting story, and from the overweight lady whose doctor gave her an Rx for patience. The envisioned prospect of your long-term goal of good solid health is the best motivator for accomplishing short-term goals. You know what you can comfortably do today. Tomorrow, up the ante a little. Little by little, as your heart, lungs, muscles, and circulatory system respond, you feel better and brighter, and you're lighter on your feet. Others will notice, but even more important, your mirror will whisper nice things. Relish the justified attention you receive and use it to boost your well-deserved pride.

Motivation

Perhaps man, having remade his environment,
will turn around at last and begin to remake himself.
Will Durant

There is no end to the better in you.

Those who search . . . find,
those who don't try . . . whine.

Self-motivation is the spark that ignites learning, doing, helping and sharing. Positive self-motivation feeds the power to dig down deep and make you better than yesterday.

A more academic definition of motivation is: "Motivation is the creation of determination," which activates a purposeful life. The definition goes on to state; good motivation moves you toward your own edification. Simply, motivation is anything that gets you off your backside to get things done. Self-motivation is the key to a bright future.

After I finished a lecture to a retirement group, a dubious lady asked me why an 87-year-old had to lose weight, get her girlish figure back and be able to move with grace and agility. I gave her all the usual reasons: she would most likely live longer when she got in shape, enhance her quality of life, increase her mental acuity, and decrease the likelihood she would fall. "With all this added health", I said, "she could more actively share herself with her family and friends. She was unimpressed. "I have all that," she said, "great-grandchildren, and I can keep up with them . . . most of the time. And I go to church and out with the girls. Isn't that enough?"

I had known her husband and felt confident to pull out my ace card and said, "With your permission, I'll give you a direct and honest response. Your husband was a great man but the reality is that he died 12 years ago. In those 12 years, have you ever thought of dating?" She replied honestly, "Yes, many times, but my time has passed and besides, who wants an old lady anyway?" I looked her right in the eyes and firmly said, "You have not passed till you have passed."

She got the point. I added, "Yes, you are 87, but you have the vitality age of about 60. You are full of spirit and creativity. And you look older than 60 because you are overweight by at least 70 pounds. Pity those poor pallbearers carrying all that extra fat." That last sentence really put the point across.

She looked at me hard and long. "I'll think about it." Fifteen seconds later she grabbed my arm and whispered in my ear, "Oh hell, you're right, how do I get started?"

Wow, that was it for me! I learned that revitalizing a long-desired goal is invigorating. It is never too late. I thought later, I'll tell her that if and when she's ready to chase a man or any other passion, she will have the agility, the power, and the endurance to do it with gusto.

And if chasing a man is not in her future, she will always know, till her dying breath, that she could have chased one if she had wanted to.

Many of us over 70 were born long before most people understood the health benefits of personal lifestyle responsibility. It is no exaggeration to say that many of today's elderly are overly dependent on their clergy, physicians, spouses, government and/or trust that God will provide. Without tested, up-to-date advice, they often falter unless they learn to prevent what was once accepted as an age-related disability. Taking charge of your own life is the first big step toward true health.

Prevention is the mantra for this 21st century. A healthy lifestyle is prerequisite to a high-quality physical, psychological and social life. But childhood attitudes often persist. There is good news, though: the over-70 population is the largest group now joining health clubs. Three cheers for personal responsibility. Old dogs do learn new tricks. A good trick is a healthy life style. There is hope.

Obesity is a good example of a faulty lifestyle. Sixty six percent of the American population is overweight or obese. There is hope, if we see the problem and do what is necessary. If an obese person loses 100 pounds, his or her quality of life is greatly enhanced. Amazingly, even the loss of just the first 10 pounds makes a huge difference in many physiological and psychological factors. As the rest of the useless fat drops off, more benefits accrue.

And the benefits pile up. Some are, more easily tying your shoes, trimming toe nails, picking things up from the floor, working in the flower beds, etc. A most important fact is the more excess weight you carry, the more stress is placed on ankles, knees, hips and back. Ignorance of how good health feels can thwart the vision of what excellent health is. Successful weight losers joyfully experience the fantastic nature of vigorous health.

The American College of Sports Medicine advises that a person lose no more than a kilo a week. A kilo is 2.2 pounds. Some calculations. There are seven days in a week and 3500 calories in a pound of fat. To achieve your lose of a kilo a week, you must shed 1200 calories a day. If that is too much, muster your patience and cut back a bit less. The trick is to eat a little less and exercise a little more. The right food and portion size, along with an, 'I can' attitude, and it can happen. Your health future is worth talking to a nutritionist and increasing your exercise, Walking around the block will allow you to keep track of the neighbors. Shoot for 10,000 steps a day. A pedometer keeps you in reality.

Garrison Keillor, the homespun Minnesota philosopher, ends his weekly, mythical Lake Wobegon radio monologue with, "Where all the women are strong, the men are good-looking and all the children are above average." You too can be from Garrison Keillor's Lake Wobegon where I might paraphrase:

everyone is strong, all are good looking, and all of us children are healthy and fit.

A new lifestyle can change your very core.
Do what you can, then a little bit more.

Optimum Health

Admittedly, it is difficult to change long-held habits. But the chances of success increase with realistic goals. Continually affirm what you want for yourself, such as decreased medical expense, more happiness, and more vitality. Short-term success is more assured when the long-term goal is optimum health.

Optimum health maximizes the functioning of muscles, bones, lungs, organs, as well as the vascular and nervous systems i.e., every cell in the body. And don't leave out the spirit. Your spirits soar when you feel great. Also, optimum health integrates all our body's systems, which gives you an exuberant glow.

Let's look at what fitness means for the following eight body systems.

Bone health maintains life-long bone strength, i.e., density.

Muscle health gives you strength and flexibility sufficient to deal with daily living and those ubiquitous emergencies.

Lung health permits greater endurance through optimum oxygen uptake by every cell in the body.

Organ health is every cell doing its job in a timely manner.

Vascular health refers to open, flexible arteries and veins functioning to transport nutrients and oxygen to all parts of the body, then returning to the lungs to reoxygenate the blood.

Nervous system health allows supervisory control of all central and automatic nerve function, such as breathing, as well as of high-level thought processes.

Spiritual health assures an ever-increasing awareness and understanding of all earthly matters and their relationship to the eternal.

System health materializes when all the above elements function for the good of the whole person and in relation to the whole community.

Research tells us that a lifestyle change that, for example, lowers overall cholesterol, pays off in a higher quality of life. Even a slight improvement in health is a powerful motivating force, which can heighten willpower. Willpower can then explode into that get-up-and-go that feels so good and gets things done. I like to drive this point home with:

> *Our total self is so complex and interrelated, that when one part of the body is made better, all other parts respond positively. Thus, a working knowledge of biological facts allows insightful common sense to become a major factor in your journey toward a healthier life.*

Genes and Exercise

An article by Frank Booth, "*Waging War on Modern Chronic Diseases: Primary Prevention through Exercise Biology,"* in the American Psychological Society Report, 2001, states that:

Physical activity triggers a gene expression pattern
that primarily promotes health.
In turn, this activated gene expression becomes self-evident
as enhanced physical performance.

Booth states that our genetic make-up is responsible for approximately 50 % of our health condition. The other 50 % stems from our lifestyle decisions. No wonder sedentary people are ill more often than active people. Even if it were possible for two persons to have the same genes, the active person would be healthier. Enhancing your gene function via exercise is just another reason to keep active.

Apathy is sometimes called *the rockin' chair syndrome.* Now we refer to this phenomenon as the couch-potato syndrome or sedentary-ism. When lack of exercise is added to an attitude of defeatism, our muscles grow weak and our nerves impotent. And, as Booth suggests, our genes give up a bit when we are sedentary. But we have the power to activate them to do their best.

As the body slows down with age and disease, the fear of falling and poor lifestyle choices increase the possibility of depression. Depression is a recognized state of grief. The usual sequence of grief is *denial, anger, bargaining, depression, and acceptance.* All but the last stage increases the likelihood of falling. Acceptance of the fact of falls brings about a search for prevention. (Advice: If someone gives a fall party, don't attend.)

A big step is the acceptance of the fact that we are not what we used to be. Our job is to keep on a-truckin', pushing ourselves, giving ourselves appropriate challenges, even though we are not what we used to be.

Debilitating neurological loss can be interpreted as loss of one's youth. That personal loss can drive your to grief. If and when you accept aging as a fact, you can get on with your life. Facing facts is a way to start gaining health information, and becoming more fit. In fact, as physical fitness increases, your physiological age can be considerably reduced. However, realistically, our biology is ultimately designed to give in, give up and give out. But until that time, know that self-sabotaging decisions can hurt you. You have the privilege to make decisions that help you live longer and have a higher quality of life. Prevention is cheaper, providing the magnificent benefit of longer independent mobility.

The organization, 50-Plus: Life Long Fitness Alliance, launched by Stanford University Physicians and Physiologists, initiated a study entitled, *The Economic Cost of Physical Inactivity.* It contains information on the actual costs of: Obesity, Diabetes, Congestive Heart Failure, Hip Fractures, and Depression. All of these, along with other chronic conditions, are aggravated by a sedentary life style.

Here is an example with regard to hip fractures. Walking two to three hours per week results in a 23% lower risk of hip fracture. There are approximately 311,000 new hip fractures reported each year in the United States. The current cost of treating a hip fracture averages

$81,000 dollars. The money is high but also considered is the cost of societal disruption due to disability. Proper conditioning exercise could reduce falls by 23%, which would save $5.8 billion. Balance refuses to add to the problem.

> Note: The organization that initiated the mentioned costs study can be found at www.50plus.org Try their site for good fitness information. Also, North Carolina has done a great deal in calculating economic costs of physical inactivity. See www.beactivenc.org/mediacenter/economicreport.cfm

Too many people deny the neurological fact that we begin to go downhill by the age of 30. The older we become, the faster we deteriorate. Denial never gets anyone anywhere. The goal of KAT is high-level neurological functioning for as long as possible. There is a lot that can be done to slow the downhill slide.

Muscle strength is one of those things. Our muscles are the most abundant tissue in the body, which makes them the largest repository of a variety of key substances. For this reason and others, loss of muscle can actually weaken the immune system. Strength training increases muscle mass that increases strength, and at the same time boosts immune system viability.

Anyone who has worked in a factory will appreciate this story. My Uncle Henry was a sly man. I worked with him for a whole week on a repetitive factory task when I was 16. Uncle Henry rarely stopped working. At mid-morning he said, "Don, would you like to take a rest?" Then he quickly said, "While we're resting let's lift that wash tub and put it over there." Please know that washtub was full to the brim with liquid. Wow, at the time I thought his definition of resting was a little perverted. Later, I discovered Uncle Henry's wisdom. Resting can consist of doing something different from your previous task. Changing from one repetitive task to another activity requires different muscles to be used, and gives us a rest of sorts. This is the principle of cross training. We have all heard the phrase, "Variety is the spice of life."

The trick is to keep on exercising till the day we die. Till the day of death? Yes, this is no exaggeration. Some one said the Grim Reaper couldn't catch you if you keep moving. Trips to the bathroom are not enough. Find a form of exercise that you like, and can practice for the learning inherent in it. You are not working for perfection; you are working to become better, both in brain and body.

Some people like yo-yos or juggling or dancing or bowling or a million other activities that require the body to move and the mind to solve learning problems. Keep goals alive, love the sweat, and reap the benefits.

Physical activity becomes a positive addiction because it makes you feel so good. You feel good because you are more fit. There are three criteria for a positive addiction. They are: *legal, healthy,* and *inexpensive.* The last is relative to what you can afford. No one can afford an unhealthy life.

It feels terrific to know that good health can cost so little. In the process, you are permitted to become your own doctor, prescribing healthy behavior. You are also your own patient, reaping the benefits.

Read on for more reasons to exercise.

Health Goals for Public Health

We all can benefit from knowing the overall picture, which is here summarized from my reading of public health goals.

1. Reduce the present disease rate by half via lifestyle changes, mainly through exercise, better nutrition, weight management, stress control, and smoking cessation. Remember, exercise brightens what apathy dampens. Physiological research has proven that reduction of illness by 50% is probably a low estimate. Your body will respond to a good life style by becoming healthier. For goodness sake, give each and every cell in your body what it needs to function well.

2. Doctors and health professionals need to publicly model their conviction that prevention of disease is vital to reducing financial costs and human suffering. However, many health workers are overweight, placing themselves in the path of inevitable disease. They are not modeling what they preach.

3. Education of the public begins with the professional's commitment to his or her specialty. But now we know how to prevent many diseases. Physicians could easily issue meaningful, officially written prescriptions for exercise. Here's a story of the reverse. A patient went into a walk-in clinic for a persistent cold. He encountered an obese MD. The doctor prescribed the appropriate medicine for the patient, then the patient wrote an exercise prescription for the doctor. The doctor read it and laughed nervously, then said, "Thanks, you're right".

A cure is not prevention, but prevention is a cure. Cures costs much more than prevention. Cure can never do any more than retain the health status quo. Prevention can quickly make our world much healthier. However, at the present time, a large percentage of the public either doesn't know or doesn't believe the power that exercise has in stacking the deck toward extraordinary health benefits. Be good to yourself and make fitness your goal.

After reading information on genetics, I began searching for metaphors to help me gain a greater depth of understanding of exercise in relation to gene-induced health activation. Play with this one. Contrast a dull, dingy, and uncared-for home with how it appears after receiving a sprucing up by a gifted designer. In the same way, even the first few pounds of weight loss feels good and noticeably improves physiological functioning. . . and looks!

The Centers for Disease Control and Prevention have found that due to physical inactivity, approximately 250,000 U.S. deaths per year occur prematurely. If you are as fiscally tight as I am, here's another fact. According to Booth, "Physical inactivity potentiates at least 17 unhealthy conditions at the cost of about $1 trillion/year." He continues, "The Center for Disease Control and Prevention has concluded, "Physical inactivity is one of the major underlying causes of premature mortality in the U.S."

Across the board, moderate physical activity would reduce the need for medical services by *half* or more. Doctors would then be free to practice the art of patience in every office visit. I can't wait.

The Spirit of Motivation

Thus far, we have learned that genes, exercise, nutrition, stress management, and lifestyle choices influence optimum health. Now, how do we get motivated to make these choices, and what are some of the pitfalls?

Often, we suffer from the consequences of many daily choices that cause misery, expense and disability. Better choices promote better outcomes. We have been allowed the custodial privilege of our very own personal bio-temple. It is a sacred piece of work, a work always in progress. We are exceedingly delicate and yet, remarkably strong at the same time. There are universal rules that dictate our procedures of care. On a practical level, these rules tell us to wear a seat belt, put on a helmet when playing football or riding a motorcycle, have several grab bars in the bathroom and a railing on stairs, avoid sunburns and debilitating stress, and refuse to exercise too little or too much. Just right is just right.

As you will learn in the next chapter, your brain is a biological jewel of galactic proportions. Your brain is so important that you have a duty and obligation to meticulously nurture it. Every construction worker knows why he or she wears a hard hat. Become practically hard headed when taking meticulous care of your brain and it will serve you well.

Good health avoids an insidious use of drugs. Illegal drugs are a flagrant violation of good biological care. Even most prescription drugs, as well as over-the-counter drugs used incorrectly, have their negative side effects. Also, the wrong combination of drugs can injure organs and the brain. Lesson: use drugs rightly and sparingly, and always under a doctors supervision.

Eating too much or too little food produces obesity or anorexia; both are no-nos. Tobacco usage, even second hand smoke, is unhealthy. Extremes in any form are counterproductive to the vigorous biological health you deserve. The opposite of extremes was offered to us by the Greeks. They spoke of *moderation in all things,* an excellent prescription for good health. The Greeks also said to *Know Thyself.* Between these two, you will find a healthful balance.

Yes, such things as genetic diseases, and structural abnormalities exist. Whatever cross you may bear, you can be thankful that you're alive --- alive is good. Our task is to be healthfully diligent with what we have been given and enjoy the journey. Healthy lifestyle choices are difficult to make, at first, but very soon, the benefits are felt and seen. Remember that sweat-producing exercise is a choice that requires persistence. If you aren't persistent, that is a choice for ill health. Occasional frustration is part of any on-going journey, but a positive mental attitude sweeps the path ahead.

Enjoying daily chores can be a profoundly religious act. Knowing that the spiritual realm is all-encompassing is helpful for us to find the joy in the life we live. A healthy body, mind, and spirit render us capable of radiant joy. A healthier life style can become your motivational escalator lifting you to a higher form of spirituality.

Progressing from your present skill level to a higher one requires practice, which is undergirded by persistence. Thus, motivation for change is a vital component of good practice.

But there is more. Putting ourselves on a solid *emotional* basis requires commitment, *social* support, and even passion. Motivation to be *moral* demands a proactive belief in fairness and justice. Beyond morality is *spirituality*, which takes us beyond thought, then paradoxically, back to ourselves. However, without durable and *physical* strength, there is no foundational basis for the good mental, social, emotional, moral, or spiritual health. Self-renewal demands diligence and persistence, which is embedded in free will.

Persistent Motivation versus Habitual Apathy

The eight factors below are gleaned from the many writings concerning those people stuck in self-defeating modes of behavior when it comes to physical exercise. These factors include:

lack of motivation
lack of a knowledge of health facts
lack of a close personal health example
lack of an affirmative philosophy
lack of a positive mental attitude
lack of personal, positive, and persistent human support
lack of willpower
lack of imagination (or experience) of how it feels to be fully healthy.

Motivation was a topic for discussion over a hundred years ago, by the psychologist, William James. He wrote that the foundation of motivation (determination) is activated by four forces of the mind. They are *attention* (focus) which gives rise to *intention* (direction). These two are joined by the compelling intensity of *volition.* Attention, intention, and volition are now combined, becoming the power of *will.* These four foundational concepts can help us understand the nature of the determination that is the meat of motivation. Willpower may be activated by intending to go for what you want, giving the matter attention and passionately demanding that you do what you want done.

For many people self-motivation seems to be a lost cause. And it is difficult to become truly independent after a long, dependent childhood. Admittedly, even though change is a universal constant, it is hard to change our habits. But change we must, where our health is concerned.

A good beginning question is, where does the motivation to change come from? The answer is in the mind, but also from knowledge, metaphors, authority figures, insights, and common sense, and who is to say that it can't come from out of this world? Before we finish, we shall talk about each of these. Let's jump right in.

The human body evolved in the dog-eat-dog period of our prehistory. Work hard or die was the norm; there was no retirement. Now leap to our sedentary modern age of computers, TV, and cheap, fatty food. No wonder our country has a problem meeting everyone's health needs.

On average, we live longer because of clean water, proper sewage disposal, and vaccines. But obesity, chronic diseases, and a reluctance to keep fit and control diet all play havoc with our quality of life, our balance included.

No one is suggesting we go back to the time when tigers ran loose. What is strongly suggested, however, is to understand that our bodies work optimally only when we do our part. The saying "Use it or lose it" is true. An optimum lifestyle includes daily challenges for agility, balance, coordination, strength training, aerobics for the heart and lungs, and joint flexibility. Don't forget that a positive mental attitude is also a part of an optimum lifestyle. Remember Johnny Mercer. "You gotta ac-cent-u-ate the positive, eliminate the negative, and don't mess with mister in between".

All efforts made toward good health work to better integrate the nervous system. A seamless body and mind generate a more intact relationship between our independence and our social responsibility. Physical zest and a hardy spirit are worthy goals.

Those prehistoric relatives of ours must have had a great will to survive. We would not be here without their strength. They did not worry about odor, sweat, and appearing unkempt. Our forebears took baths under the local waterfall. Luckily, these days, every gym has a shower with your name on it.

This next section approaches motivation from many different angles. At least one will reach deep into your brain and speed you toward better balance and health. Choose one or two that you like and give it all you have.

The Lick Factor

I was amazed to learn that no one had named a universal phenomenon. I call it *The Lick Factor.* It is the basis of the KAT axiom "Do what you can, then a little bit more." Here's a couple of examples. This idea came to me when I was licking an ice cream cone. My question was how many licks does it take to devour one dip? The point: do a little at a time, stay with it, and reap the benefits. Little by little and you get a lot.

A more practical example involves our American cars. If every driver would drive a car with just a little greater gas efficiency, we would quickly become independent of most foreign oil. Another example is if we turned off just one 100-watt light bulb for an hour a day, we would need fewer power plants. Also, a rarely known fact is that little appliance light that is on 24/7 adds up to five percent of our U.S. power usage. Do we need to have that appliance on all the time? The point is that even an infinitesimal amount of individual effort multiplied by the millions soon adds up. This is especially true with human progress toward changing for the better.

Self-motivation is based on a powerful force called personal responsibility. As you progressively become your own balance coach, you and you alone decide just what and how much more you do each day. Obviously, physical balance is enhanced by your mental ability to power your will. Start small, stay with it and healthy progress will follow.

The KAT Axiom

The above Lick Factor promoted the creation of the KAT axiom, which is:

Do what you can, then a little bit more.

Apply this axiom to your balance quest. You perform literally millions of thoughts, decisions, and motor transactions each day. When each of your neurological transactions is made a tiny bit more efficient, you will find your progress toward health goes faster. Your loved ones will wonder what miracle happened. You may even surprise yourself. A better tomorrow is assured when many "littles" come together as improved functioning.

Let yesterday be your guide while using today as your time bridge to tomorrow's goals. You don't have to be a perfectionist, but you must have some idea of where you want to go and the action needed to take you there.

Here is a four line Rapp rap that looks at the concept of *little* using a rap beat.

A little bit of this and a little bit of that.
Variety of movement, now that's where it's at.
The brain gets better the more you move.
You folks reading this are in the right groove.

Both muscles and nerves require small increments of challenge each day to keep their strength and integrity. Become your own balance coach by setting out a schedule of exercise. Just plain walking is a good challenge for the heart, vascular and lung health, and especially balance. Plainly, start with what you can do comfortably. Then increase the intensity and distance as you become more fit. When you become progressively more fit you become more comfortable with daily chores and actually extend your life.

All learning benefits from the KAT axiom, *Do what you can then a little bit more.* It has such nice meter I added three more lines. I love to delude myself into thinking Tennyson would have liked it.

Do what you can then a little bit more.
If you don't do your best you're an absolute bore.
Do what you can then a little bit better,
And someday you'll be an Irish Setter.

Note: A psychiatrist once told me that the best layman definition of mental and physical health was *bright eyed and bushy-tailed.* An Irish Setter serves well as the model for this image. Irish Setters are clear eyed, eager, frisky, tail-wagging examples of vitality and vigor. Wouldn't it be nice to get what they've got? It's possible.

The KAT motto is a self-protective device. It requires each class member to become responsible for his or her own safety and progress. There is no way for the instructor of a group to be 100% responsible for everyone. The motto sends a message well beyond the class, of being responsible for the self at any time and any place. Responsibility keeps you more alert, and that's good when it comes to avoiding the pot holes in life.

Here are three suggestions that heighten personal responsibility:

- Realistically acknowledge your present physical and mental realities.
- Learn the reasons *why* your body, regardless of age or disability, can do better than it presently does.
- Make decisions on *how* much more you can do each day. These decisions should always be made with safety in mind.

Know that lifestyle changes require some adjustment time. Best to begin slowly, gaining momentum as you go, and soon you will feel age-related changes.

Robert Redford, the actor lends active assistance to budding film directors through his Sundance Film Festival for independent films. He echoes KATs axiom with his statement, "If you can do more, you should". I love succinct when it is so nice and brief.

Eager Beavers, Goals and Affirmations

Teaching an adult class is extremely rewarding. Wonderful things happen. Here's a story of an eager beaver 75-year-old class member. His age is made obvious by his gnarled face and sparse gray hair. Everyone reacts to him with an expressive "Oh my, what a man!" Many ask him his secret. He gives them the orthodox response, such as, "Must be my genes," or "I take after my 100-year-old mother." But in private, he was deadpan as he pointed his finger at me. "I'll tell you my secret if you promise not to tell anyone in class." "Of course," I said. By this time, I really did not know what to expect. He said he often repeated these two lines to himself:

> "I'm eager as a beaver, I work like a dog.
> My everyday habit is to think like a rabbit."

Notice he did not say to behave like a rabbit. Specifically, the very act of thinking exciting thoughts indicates you're still alive. We giggled a bit then he said, "You can use it in your book as long as you don't use my name." He joked, "I share this with you because you love 'fabulous poetry'. Then he got to the serious part. "Even more, you understand the power of personal affirmational statements and their positive influence on health." I sensed it was my turn to say something. "Yes, we say positive and/or negative things to ourselves all the time. Your little poem is playing out the idea of Johnny Mercer's lyrics. Remember his 1940s song, "Ac-cen-to-ate the Positive"? My eager-beaver friend said, "Don, when I think of a Johnny Mercer song, all I can think of are the Andrew sisters."

> Note: this is the second mention of a Mercer song. I loved the lyrics in the 40"s and still think of them with their affirmational force. Also, the first line was not sung as it is spelled. Rather it was sung ac-cent---chuate.

His story highlights the fact that the linguistic part of ourselves can influence all the rest of us. Words are thoughts and both are powerful, and together they work wonders. Our self-talk is obviously very personal. What we choose to call positive is very important business.

Goals as a Motivational Tool

My eager-beaver, work like a dog class member obviously benefits from his "poetic" self-talk. His high level of fitness is his proof. His little poem was his way to move himself off his dime toward a dollar's worth of wellness.

But goals are a little different. Let's focus on the steps to formulate meaningful goals. First, a silly question: How do you climb a ladder? The obvious answer is, one rung at a time. Without each rung, we would never reach the top. Each rung is a short-term goal in pursuit of a long-term goal. Achieving your goals is analogous to climbing a ladder one rung at a time. Someone once said, "I did not know where I was going till I started out for somewhere else." Merely to move up one rung allows a better view of the possibilities.

Another student, a successful professional man of 55, wanted to roller-blade. He knew it was dangerous for him. He had never before been active in sports and admitted he was more than flabby. My first response, "You do know you can live a perfectly happy life and never roller-blade." But he wanted to learn and goals are to be respected. Difficult goals are possible, as long as you climb toward them one rung at a time.

His genius was that he understood the ladder analogy. He needed to crawl before skating. He needed to become fit, speed up his reaction time, and increase his agility and coordination. Also, he needed to learn to roller-skate first, which is a lot easier than roller-blading. He understood his reality. Nothing good comes in an instant. Patience is part of the formula. Exhaustive preparation was needed for a skill that could have been extremely dangerous for an over weight and awkward 55-year-old man.

Now I let him have the serious part of this. " I said, "Here's another test of your reality. Let's imagine that you never fully learn to roller-blade. But in the meantime, you become fit, people notice that you are firmer, you feel better and have more energy, and you've learned to roller-skate and enjoy it. Look what the long-term goal of roller-bladding has done for you. You were motivated to follow a healthy routine long enough to change your physiology, your posture, your appearance, and you achieved an enjoyment level in a new and challenging activity." Then I added, "All elements in a good fitness routine have physical, mental, emotional, and social benefits." He got the point.

The attainment of most of our goals is rooted first in motor fitness; especially balance, which is basic to our well-being and independence. Second, both mental and physical fitness form the foundation of bio-movement defined as life.

Now for the rest of his story. He did not fully learn to enjoy roller-blading, but his fitness level did increase notably. He also took pleasure in the fact that he had tried. Now he goes to the skating rink often, which is a 180-degree change from his previous more sedentary life. Rome was not built in a day. That's why short-term diets rarely work for long-term needs.

Think of the Lick factor when you begin anything. Chip away at the task and it will be complete. Patience is King. Over a hundred years ago Goethe said it this way:

Whatever you can do or dream you can do begin it.
Boldness is genius, power and there's magic in it.
Only engage and the mind grows heated.
And then the task will be completed.
Goethe

The Wiggle Philosophy

Teaching University students was my life for 34 years. My *wiggle universe* lecture was one of my favorites in Child Development. Students commented that it was humorous yet a serious way to state that movement is life, and life is most evident in self-initiated movement. The opposite of movement is the state of rigor mortis and you don't want that. Too often, the ability to move freely is only understood as precious after it is drastically diminished or lost. To wiggle means to get off the couch and do something useful. An Irish Setter wiggles his whole backside.

Growth

This wiggle philosophy leads to solid growth. It suggests the obvious, that a little wiggle, or squiggle, or ripple, can grow into a big wave. Witness a baby, given time, becomes an adult. For all of us, short-term goals are stepping-stones to the achievement of long-term goals. But the reverse is also true. Long-term goals can often be the catalyst to activate short-term goals. These two are much more than two peas in a pod; they are the peas and the pod as well as the roots, the soil, and the rain. Leave any of these elements out and you have no growth at all.

My KAT growth goal for you is to gain motor fitness to the point that you never fall. If Kinetic Arts Training, along with your effort, prevents just one fall related injury, it is worth it. A large percentage of older people who break their hips from a fall never get out of a wheelchair. Worse, some of those people die from their first fall. I repeat, just one hip fracture costs, on average, $81,000. If those fallers had been in good physical condition, many may have avoided the fall with quicker reactions and stronger muscles. A good portion of the present cost, of 5.8 billion dollars, could be saved. Good balance is well worth making preventive efforts. Besides, good overall health reduces pain and anguish, and all because of your proactive stance as your own agent of prevention.

Another suggestion. At each stage of the goal achievement process, be satisfied; i.e., celebrate even the tiniest bit of improvement. We do a lot of good things for others and ourselves and no one knows what we do. The point is, if you don't praise yourself, you will never reap the benefits promoted by rightfully earned appreciation. We need that zestful feeling to re-energize ourselves, to eagerly move toward the next achievement level. I even make this point to elementary school children, but with them I add, "Only praise yourself for good things." Some of the younger ones are still struggling with what is good.

Ten Aspects of Goal Achievement

Affirmations are statements that prepare your mind for achieving the next goal. Goals are statements of what is wanted. Affirmation readies your mind for attacking the goal with dedication and gusto. Use the following ten suggestions to formulate both goals and affirmations.

- State your goals *positively*. Continually move toward your goal, never run from it.
- Make your goals *personal.* Vividly demand your own undivided attention.
- State your goals in the *present tense. Now* is where you live.
- Make each goal *reachable*. Insist on one fruitful and successful step at a time.
- Make your goals *specific*. See them with exactness and clarity.
- Write your goals. Words on paper possess particular potency.
- Make goals *brief.* Make them sharp and to the point.
- *Repeat* your goals many times a day, especially early in the morning and late at night.
- Goal achievement requires *personality changes*. Tomorrow's self deserves more than yesterday's warmed-over self.
- Make goals *rhyme*, (if you can,) Rhyme and meter make them memorable and more fun to repeat.

A metaphor: A bullet is placed in the rifle chamber. The eye, guided by a brain, sights and aims the gun barrel toward the target, and a finger pulls the trigger. The shell is designed to explode, sending the bullet at unimagined speed down the barrel to the target.

Let's use Gestalt Therapy to interpret the motivational aspect of this metaphor. Imagine that you are the bullet, packed with an explosive emotional charge. You are also the barrel as well as the trigger. You are the brain and eyes that sight the target. Your finger pulls the trigger. You are even the target who is the aim of all your effort.

This type of focused thinking makes your motivation become more intimate and personal. You are the object of your own action as well as the totality of the process. Your lifestyle is the process and you are the goal. You are the only one on your rifle range. This is a one-person show. You are even the audience, who is always somewhere watching and can praise or criticize your performance. This type of thinking puts the word RESPONSIBILITY in all caps. The following ten-word affirmation is most apt:

If it is to be, it is up to me.

The great American philosopher and radio comedian, Fred Allen, once quipped, "You only live once, but if you live it right, once is enough!" Living right is being fit and healthy in order to better help yourself and others.

I repeat Buckminster Fuller's two marvelous lines that highlight a serious reason to take care of yourself.

The environment to each must be. . . everything that isn't me.
The Universe in turn must be . . . everything that isn't me . . . plus me.
Fuller

You and I are important parts of the universe. We all share responsibility to make it work. If anyone has ever called you dumb or stupid, he or she was ignorant of our inherent universal connection. Thinking big is healthy.

Here is another metaphor. Picture a local sports bar on Saturday night after the local team loses badly. Sad bunch of fans. Just then, a nationally recognized, handsome, charismatic, debonair sports figure bursts in with a gorgeous woman hanging on each arm. The women in the room are shaken from their depression by their desire to be on his arm and the men are invigorated by their desire for his fame, his money, his ability, and his women.

The point: amazing transformations can happen, lifting us from gloom to high spirits. Exercise is one of those transforming agents. It wakes up genes, and in turn the activated genes help us function better. Everyone benefits when participation in health enhancement is pervasive. You want insurance rates to come down? Refuse to get sick. As individuals direct more effort to prevention, all health costs will come down. Exercise initiates a flood of chemistry surging to the brain that enlivens, brightens, and promotes sound thinking. Try it, you'll like it.

Eight Steps to Action

Psychologist James Bugental has suggested an eight-step progression to get things done. Knowing these steps will help you nurture a weak idea into a worthwhile outcome. The first step is *intention.* Intention is a bubble-like thought rising from the unconscious. The action of a wish can render a bubble more solid. The *wish* can progress into a *want*, and on to a *desire*. Only then is desire energized into the power of *will.* If there is enough willed intensity, *action* follows. And, if enough strength is generated by action, it *actualizes* into an *interaction*. And as Goethe says," then the task will be completed". Omit any one of these steps and the original intention remains a foggy dream.

> Note: There is a remarkable similarity between Bugental's formulation and William James's four elements of Mind: intention, attention, volition and will.

Too many of us become rocking-chair minded, depressed, unconcerned, detached, dejected, downhearted, blue, and despondent. What a heck of a list! Even one of those is unhealthy. However, there is an action antidote called *purpose*. Admittedly, it is difficult to pull purpose out of thin air because even finding a purpose must go through the intention to interaction process. This process can take a very short time or perhaps a lifetime. Conscious attention to the Bugental process will assure that the process completes its journey to success. A life of quality is the process of beginning small and becoming what you will. Here are Bugental's eight listed with a little more detail.

> *Intention* breaks through to consciousness and becomes a wish
> *Wish* is very weak, but when nurtured becomes a want.
> *Want* focuses a wish into a desire
> *Desire* heightens the power of will.
> *Will* bridges the gap between thought and action.
> *Action* is that first directed movement toward actualization.

Actualization is a deed, word, or process that generates interaction.
Interaction is the outgrowth of the intention-interaction process.

There is no guarantee that the product of your interaction will bear healthy fruit. But nothing ventured nothing gained. Remember it all begins with a good intention.

The Power of Hope and Expectation

Hope and expectation are:

street sweepers clearing the road ahead. And/or
the words that soften uncertainty and untangle confusion. And/or
the sports drink, multiplying energy and heightening bulldog persistence.

Play this word game with me. Spell out the word *h o p e* vertically. Notice the restrictions placed on choosing the defining words.

Health is Highly Healing.
Openness to Optimism nurtures Optimum Opinions.
Positive Patience pervades Persistent Purpose.
Enliven your Enthusiasm with Earthy Exercise.

Try the above method for any word or concept that you want to drive deep into your mind. Define each letter in any way you want. This thought-word game helps to broaden your thought process and at the same time clarify your thinking. Each letter of H O P E now becomes a motivating element.

Hope is more than optimism. Naive optimism says that everything will be okay, but levelheaded hope accepts reality with open eyes and mind. This practical kind of hope engenders a realistic expectation that life is life until it isn't. Hope is the courage to take risks, along with the common sense to minimize the dangers of risk. Without hope, the likelihood of acting on your own behalf is out of the question. The elderly need hope and expectation more the most. Death is closer for them than it is for their children or grandchildren. A healthy older person knows the facts of biology, and acts accordingly.

Hope is explicitly expressed in the KAT philosophy. Hope is the precursor of motivational intent. Hope is embedded in the reality of the future. Poetically, both expectation and hope bring up the sun after a long winter's night. Perspicacity, persistence, and goal setting are their outcome. Sweat is part of healthy hope as much as it is part of healthy body functioning. Hope is palatable and nourishing in its texture and tone. It tastes, smells and feels great when even an infinitesimal speck of hope is perceived. Hope is the path to the next step, the next therapy or next practice, the next workday, the next confession, and the next success.

Hope, says William James, is that mental state of mind that is activated by body action. He advised that if you want to be happy, do something happy. Today's medical and psychological communities have found James to be unerring when he links mental states with bodily action. Our mental state follows bodily action and vice versa. We become what we do as we progress to what we will become.

The body and brain are indivisible. We are a total unity. Our body-brain is a galaxy of inter and inner connections and potentials. We have possibilities beyond what we can reason, and strangely enough, we do not yet fathom how great we really are. Witness the immigrant who begins with nothing and achieves beyond anyone's dream. Wonder is part of hope. Then the next step is to wonder about your wonder. After all, how in the heck are you ever going to become wonderful if you can't wonder about anything and everything?

And last, hope, expectation, and wonder are fraternal triplets. They may not be spelled alike, but they come from the same womb of optimism. Your job is to find that source, because these triples are continually reborn when fed with curiosity or awe. You might then be eligible to join KAT's Optimists Club. Its charter members were, you guessed it, expectation, wonder, curiosity, awe and especially hope. Your job is cut out for you. Begin each day with the poet Blake at your side, saying, I hold infinity in the palm of my hand and eternity in the next hour.

There is no way to label my positive mental attitude as pie in the sky. It is anatomically and physiologically a fact that the brain controls our cellular functions. On top of that, the brain has power to make itself better.

Pragmatically these findings offer something for everybody. Miracles do happen in very difficult cases, because our bodies and brain are more complicated, sophisticated, fabulous, and even more god-like than we understand. Every neuroscientist knows and respects the healing wisdoms of the body and mind together. Talk nicely to yourself and nice you get in return.

Positive Mental Attitude (PMA)

Your mental attitude determines how you see your world. And what you choose to see and feel makes up what your think. A glass seen as half empty reeks of pessimism, however, a glass half full accepts the opportunity to fill it.

A PMA encourages a healthy approach to all you do, and say, and think. This example will make the point. In high school I was given a list of titles for an essay we had to write. I choose, *A Silk Purse from a Sow's Ear.* I only remember that at 14, I already knew the concept. A case in point was an Aunt who wore expensive cloths, put on a lot of make up and did what I thought was a ridiculous thing to her hair. They demonstrated her wish to be a silk purse. But my Aunt was fat, flabby and huffed and puffed when she got up from a chair. Sows are more agile than she was. She was obviously taking care of her out side appearance but her insides were a mess. She died young.

However, both outside and inside need attention. Which brings up the point that challenges the half-full half empty analogy. My Aunt thought her glass was half full when she showed off expensive clothing. But she was delinquent in not seeing her unfulfilled physical health. The moral: Think in two or more dimensions. What you show is important, but so is the inside world that is the real you.

Some prominent examples of purveyors of the a positive mental attitude were Norman

Vincent Peale, Robert Schuler, Napoleon Hill, and Zig Zigler, I hasten to add all those sweet but tough grandmothers out there who coach their grandchildren with positive talk and deed. Also, remember the Dale Carnegie seminars, where his stock in trade was to encourage enthusiasm. Carnegie's glass was overflowing. Willy Loman's empty glass became his instrument of suicide. Enthusiasm is basic to a positive mental attitude. The energy of enthusiasm activates clarity of thinking that hopefully is biased in the direction of your own well being.

Need another reason to cultivate a PMA? Try this on for size. There are more than seven billion people on our planet. Each one has a unique set of cells, biological efficiencies, interests and goals. No one else is like you. That makes you very important; you are one of a kind. Fred Rogers, of *Mr. Roger's Neighborhood*, dedicated his life to the fact of every child's uniqueness. An undercurrent of his show was a message for all of us. Our childhood experience is our present attitudinal foundation, i.e. the basis of who we are. We can choose the best from our childhood, and nurture it into a positive mental attitude.

Health demands that we retain our child-like ability to grow, wonder, learn, and above all, look at the world as half full and then fill it with worthwhile choices and behavior. It is easier to do this when you know you are unique.

Ambiguity is the opposite of a PMA. Ambiguity restrains the journey to health. Ambiguity is a cross between a raging pit bull and Lassie. The pit bull chews your leg off while Lassie goes for help. Chronic ambiguity leads to discouragement. Don't go down that path. Haven't you heard, the glass is half full? Let's drink to health.

For the older set, I repeat these lines. Longfellow was right on the money when he wrote:

For age is opportunity no less than youth itself,
though in another dress.
And as the evening twilight fades away,
the sky is filled with stars . . . invisible by day.

Note: A positive mental attitude is just that, a positive interpretation of the world and your life there in.

In recent speeches, I ended my call for more fitness by saying:

"Stand up tall, suck in your gut, stick out your chest
and show the world your pride in your journey to your best. "

The moment I ended the line whole audience broke out in smiles and straightened up. The message was delivered. If this message has some relevance to you, begin with a smile.

The Rules of Change

A common-sense philosophy recognizes the *Rules of Change.* Here is a stark example. A man walked near a steep cliff. He knew a fall would kill him, but he closed his eyes and moved toward the cliff anyway. Over he went. Of course, the fall killed him. However, his death was precipitated by his decision to ignore danger. The same with drunk drivers. Under the influence, the rules of perception change. The consequences are often horrendous.

A balance class member forgot the rule of change and could have been sorely injured. He entered a large, well-known store. At the entrance was a rubber mat. The flooring became carpet, and then tile. To get the whole picture you must know that it was raining very hard. His feet were wet, and previous walkers had made the tile slippery. He reached the tile and now can't even remember hitting the back of his head on the floor. He came away with a headache, was black and blue and embarrassed for his lack of awareness. He is lucky he can still think.

His confession to me was painful. Yes, he knew the rule of change, which applies to slippery wet tile floors, but he failed to apply the rule at the right time and place. Physical circumstances such as slippery floors are to be known for what they are . . . dangerous.

The rule has many variations, depending upon the situation. *When the situation changes, the rules change.* Our balance class became more important to him, for he clearly saw it was a way to heighten his attention level along with his reaction time. He promised himself, his wife and his insurance agent that he would follow the Rules of Change from now on.

Where did the rule of change come from? It has been around as long as the Universe. I first became aware of it as the Boy Scout motto: *Be Prepared.* Part of preparedness is learning about the sequential nature of cause and effect. Part of life is being aware of eventualities. When you know the rule that says a pothole can hurt you, you prepare to avoid them.

Being prepared and staying ahead of the game is the KAT way. The goal is to skip to your grave or, better yet, dance till the music stops.

I once met Ashley Montagu, the well-known British anthropologist, at a child development meeting. He was then 73 years old, and a marvelous original thinker. He was a broadly educated man who wrote books on many subjects. He exuded vitality, insatiable curiosity, and an inspirational spirit. His memory is still ablaze in me. In a 1977 *Psychology Today* interview, Montagu said, "if you continue to *love, work, play* and *think critically*, you will not grow old as fast as when you do none of these". He was obviously living his own philosophy. Now, more than 25 years later, American College of Sports Medicine (ACSM) exercise physiologists are saying exactly the same thing. Montagu knew it from self-observation and his anthropological findings. Now we know it from experimental research, even on the cellular level. I dare to sum up Dr. Montagu as follows:

Love your work and play and think critically
on how to make your love, and work, and play ever better and better.

Appendix F paraphrases Montagu's 26 healthy childhood growing young traits. He suggests that is possible to reclaim some of your child-like vitality by 'grow young'.

Walter Bortz, M.D., says much the same thing in his book, *Die Young as Late as Possible.* Another of Bortz's book, *Dare to Be 100, where he* gives 100 strategies for retaining youthfulness into advanced age. The word *Dare* in the title means:

D - Diet - Beware of free radicals, saturated fats, etc.
A - Attitude - Make yourself necessary. Maintain your creative spark.
R - Renewal - Recharge yourself; keep working and playing.
E - Exercise - Use exercise to keep your oxygen tanks healthy.

Bortz was the keynote speaker at the American College of Sports Medicine conference in 2002 and again in 2004. The 2004 keynote title was "Disease Costs: Fitness Saves." I quote from Dr. Bortz: "The healthier we are as a person, or as a nation, the more financial resources we will generate. Health and wealth cohere. How long will it be until we learn this lesson? Have we not tried everything else already? Living longer is a choice, not fate. Living long is active, not passive. You create your own destiny." I can only add that becoming more balanced is one of the cornerstones of a quality life.

The Teacher's Story

I once asked a high school teacher how she got so much from her students. Even the "destined-to-fail" kids seemed to brighten up in her class. Please make the connection of the teacher's story to your own health and fitness quest. I paraphrase her passionate response.

I make a personal assumption that each one of my so-called failure kids appears that way because they can't see beyond their inexperienced teenage noses. Teens, like most of us, are short-term goalers. Many of them have had little hope in their lives to bolster long-term commitments. In the face of those odds, I merely assume they can and will do better.

Then I go the next step. I tell them publicly, as well as individually, that my faith in their 'hidden' value has two possible outcomes. I say: If you never come out of your self destructive, dead-end attitude you will only remember me as a pie-in-the-sky fool. I must admit I would hate that. However, if I am right, and you do have the courage to reexamine yourself for your strengths and work to throw off your self-imposed ignorance, you will remember me as a saint. You will also remember me as a person who is always on your side; on the side of your growth toward becoming a useful, productive, responsible and valuable human being.

She continued, I then add a barbed hook. If you fail to reinvent yourself and never improve, you will be even more disappointed in yourself than I will be. Why? Because we have both failed. And two negatives never make a positive. And let's be even clearer. I did not become a teacher because I wanted to be disappointed in myself.

Not through yet, she went on. "Now, a guarantee. I will be right here, and you will be right there. If we push and pull together, we can work wonders. Think about it. We are on one side, the same side, and that side is spelled Y-O-U. And the U in you stands for universe." My kids are always are puzzled by the Universe part. I explain. You are a virtual universe of possibilities. It is your lifelong task to discover your place in your universe.

When she said that, I felt as though she was pointing her finger right at me. I will remember this teacher's story for a long time

Does her type of positively biased assumption work? The research of Harvard psychologist Dr. Robert Rosenthal proves it does, as described in his book, *Pygmalion in the Classroom.* His lifetime work is based on what he calls *experimenter bias.* He has proven experimenter bias time and time again, in many different situations, with all kinds of people and even animals. When the caretaker, teacher, friend, or parent is positively biased on behalf of the other person's prospects, that person is strongly influenced in a positive direction. Under conditions of positive support, hope really does spring eternal.

What is the lesson for our quest for balance? We need to become our own caretaker, teacher, friend, parent, coach, and physician. Let's add cheerleader to the list. I suggest that KAT class members insist on being in charge of their own destiny, realistically of course, within their situational limits. You are also your own body-mind custodian, which includes being your own nutritionist, exercise trainer and minister. You write the script and design the sets and are unequivocally the most important VIP in the audience or on the stage.

If the bar you set is too low, set it just right for your own improvement schedule. To be the star of anything as important your life, you must insist on good health. Start by insisting on less fat, less caffeine, more sweat, and less wasted time. You don't have time to become addicted to anything, except your better health and what you do with it when you get it.

If you are fully satisfied with your present self, then a little part of you is already dead. Say to yourself: if I am not dead and life is about being fully alive to my complete advantage and satisfaction. That glimmer of desire to become a better person is your ticket to become the person you want to be. *There is no end to the better in your better.*

Part of your motivation can be my hopeful bias for you. Positive thoughts are lighter than a pill, more valuable than money, more potent than uranium, and a lot cheaper than *sin.* They are even cheaper than a 1930s ice cream cone. Listen to that still small voice inside your own head. I hope it tells you to read on and let KAT ideas turn you on to your own possibilities.

Zeal for Fitness

Motivation is a passion, a conviction of will. Health-oriented zeal, like religious passion, has all the elements of a powerful motivator. The three aspects of religion are: *belief, ritual,* and *ethics.* Think of these and their pertinence to your own quest for health and fitness.

Belief is:

- trust in the resiliency of biology.
- conviction in the power of your will.
- confidence in the infinite possibilities of health and well-being.

Ritual is:

- disciplined planning.
- appropriate and regular exercise and diet.
- stress management.
- rewarding relationships.

Ethics are:

- balanced responsibilities to yourself
  and all other family, public and Universal loyalties

Gibran's Prophet

Belief, ritual, and ethics are also central to Kahlil Gibran's wisdom-laden book, *The Prophet.* Since 1923, Gibran has inspired a world of thoughtful readers. He speaks poetically of your attitude toward *work*:

> You have been told also that life is darkness,
> and in your weariness
> you echo what was said by the weary.
> And I say that life is indeed darkness
> save when there is *urge*,
> and urge is blind save when there is *knowledge*,
> and all knowledge is vain save when there is *work*,
> and all work is empty save when there is *love*:
> and when you work with love
> you bind yourself to yourself,
> and to one another,
> and to God.

Work includes housework, homework, paid work . . . any work. All work requires practice to get it right. All practice is preceded by an *urge* to become better. Practice is strengthened by the *knowledge* that your goal can be accomplished. The outcome is not left to chance when what you think and do is bathed in *love.* In the process, you become better and, as Gibran says, you bind yourself to yourself. The zest for life and love is the glue. The lifelong task of becoming whole is one of pursuing the path of practice.

Through work, a person becomes whole. Work sharpened his or her wits at every stage of the process of becoming. Beginning is part of the urge, and knowledge is the strategy needed for the follow-through. Practice is the energy to refine, remake and get it right.

There always needs to be the reminder that right is what is fully right for you in relation to others and society. In your personal court of what's right, you become the judge, you are the jury, your are both lawyers, and you are the sole client. Your lifestyle quality is your judgment and your willingness to help others is your public jury. How to get to where you want to be? Suggestion: *Do what you can, then a little bit more.* (I'll bet you have heard that before.)

The above thoughts are nothing new. Remember Goethe's poem? He is also in the business *to urge* when he says:

> *Whatever you can do or dream you can do, begin it.*

Note: The complete poem is back on page 35.

Time Is Manageable

Time is a hammer, a bulldozer, and an extinguisher of suns. Biologically we flow in the river of time from the past to the present to the future. Yes, biology forces us to make our appearance in the presence of time as well as only in the present time. You can't do that when you're unaware of your place in your time. Fully awaken yourself today so you can do, ponder, learn, and design your tomorrows according to your own plan.

Practice takes time. People complain they don't have time. And that's right . . . if they say you haven't the time, you haven't. But if you say, "yes" to time, your behavior changes and you experience time in a new and expansive way. We live in time as much as in space.

Managing your time is not really a time problem; rather, it is a decision problem. When time drags, boredom blooms. Charles Tart's book, *Waking Up*, asks us to make the decision to fully wake up. Tart, a clinical psychologist, says we are too often dangerously unaware, even when we're awake. When learning a new motor skill, or revamping an old one, such as walking after a week in bed, you had better pay extraordinary attention to the task at hand.

By definition, sleep is a depressed state, which is the opposite of being unaware of reality. Buoyant health is an active, awake state. Try asking yourself this pointed wake-up question. *What is the best use of my time . . . RIGHT NOW?* The emphasis is on the right *now*. Your brain is designed to find an answer.

What you've done in the past is evident is what you are today. The here-and-now is where you reside. What you do today is the grist for tomorrow's mill. If you are apathetic, your get-up and-go-becomes slow-down-and-quit. To move on you must want more than you are today.

Here is one great remedy. Turn off that one-eyed, two-dimensional, mesmerizing world of TV. Do real things, like study and contemplate useful ideas, then share your learning with real people. Lifelong learning is a prescription for good health. And good health blossoms when you know that you have power to become more than yesterday, and better and better as time goes on.

The judicious use of your time requires a strong desire to change. That kind of energy is best driven by the power of will. However, willpower is more than an abstract topic and more than a personal trait. It also includes the biologically driven will to survive. Many of us fail to realize the power we have been given.

The question is, why aren't we more motivated to change when we "know" to think better, do better, and live better is the way to go. Self-motivation is wonderfully productive? Change requires adjustment. Each time you breathe your lungs and ribs adjust their capacity. Each time you take a step, you adjust your balance to stay in line with your center of gravity. Our motivation for making changes is very personal. Sometimes sadly, it takes a heart attack to make us move toward a healthier life style. However, the written word can also be a prime mover. And sometimes you just have to realize that the lifestyle you now lead is leading to oblivion. You are more likely to find your change trigger when you search for it.

Motivational Willingness

Motivation includes the willingness to listen, take expert direction, uncover and review health information, sweat out your daily poisons, stop doing unhealthy things, and model a lifestyle that others will flock to imitate.

Lifestyle changes are often difficult. My task is to be as motivational as possible. Some of my efforts are meant to be fun, because fun is activating. And personal thought and action are required for becoming fit, healthy and exhibiting your own style of zest.

Here are some *willingness* statements to tell yourself.

> I am willing to live fully.
> I am willing to change my lifestyle.
> I am willing to cultivate a passion for life.
> I am willing to think and talk about health.
> I am willing to do things I have not done before.
> I am willing to think in a way I have not done before.
> I am willing to sweat in the pursuit of moving forward.
> I am willing to follow my dreams toward greater health.
> I am willing to share my health enhancement with others.
> I am willing to involve myself with balance enhancement.
> I am willing to conquer frustrations and persist again and again.
> I am willing to take setbacks in stride and continue in spite of them.
> I am willing to help others toward their own motivational self-reliance.

Start this with one thought. Think of it as the first step in your health race. The process puts your on track to a "skip-to-my-Lou" exuberance.

Skip-to-my Lou" exuberance, you can't buy.
But it will come when you let your mind fly,
to the way you alone want to be.
Then success, dear friend, you will presently see.

The Brain

Our brain is the instrument, and we are the music.
The quality of our performance depends
on how we rehearse our instrument.

What do: Grandma falling down,
a persistent scientific researcher, a person in a midlife crisis,
and a successful goal achiever, have in common?
You got it, it's the *brain.*

Our brain is three pounds of magnificent, protoplasmic structure, which, as far as we know is organized as the most complicated, wonderful, productive, beautiful, and creative entity in the entire universe.

This description may be a little over the top, but no one can deny that human biology is a magnificent work in progress. It includes our nervous system, and the structural components that connect all parts of our body to each other. The central nervous system includes our brain, which connects our function to behavior, our goals to action, and our past to our present. Thanks to the myriads of partnership between our brain and our body, we are capable of planning and executing a purposeful future.

A partnership is a duality. However, the human entity requires a trinity, of sorts, in becoming more brain balanced. You must know that:

life is a *fact,*
life is an *art,*
and your life is your *future.*

The fact of human life is a progressive work of art
that is on permanent loan to a gallery called *The Future.*

Richard Restak, who wrote *Mozart's Brain and the Fighter Pilot: Unleashing Your Brain's Potential,* says that good mental faculties can be briefly summarized in three words: the ability to *attend,* to *identify,* and to *act.* These abilities are under our conscious control. We can become more alert and focused, and we can discern and function in a more purposeful manner. The sharper these three abilities are, the better we get on with our lives.

Mel Levine, M.D., in his book, *A Mind at a Time*, asks, how does the brain generate new pathways, search for thoughts, and store memories most effectively? His answer is that the brain is a pattern-searching and pattern-forming organ that stores all that it perceives. One hint at how this works is the following quotation: *"You can change your mind but you can't exchange it."* The brain knows this and performs for you alone, till death do you part. You can help your brain with its functioning by keeping healthy in body and mind. Restructuring your brain-mind is what learning is all about. A lot more on this later.

Commenting on the motor aspects of brain development, Levine states, "It turns out that a child's proficiency in sports offers one of the most transparent views of certain brain connections. Athletic progress (or its embarrassing absence) is a highly revealing gauge of gross motor performance during childhood." This is not only true for children. It is also true for any reasonably healthy brain of any age. An old dog can learn new tricks.

In his second book, *All Kinds of Minds*, Levine attends to three categories: mental energy controls, processing controls, and production controls. The word *control* is important here. The brain wants to be in control. Control is its function. But it needs help to maintain its control over a body and brain whose functions too soon decline. The answer to this age related decline is practice. Nothing earth shattering, just practice.

Dave Finnegan, a fellow juggler, has developed a practical brain-bettering program for school children. He has traveled the country for 30 years teaching elementary-school children to juggle. He has witnessed thousands of children move from complete ignorance of juggling to high-skill levels. Dave compares the novice juggler's untrained brain to an impenetrable jungle choked with undergrowth. Untrained jugglers appear awkward and ill coordinated and get lost in their own efforts.

Remarkably, little by little, the learner clears communicative trails by hacking pathways through the neural jungle. The practice process forges wider, smoother, and more easily traversed links. In a sense, the brain becomes etched with usable lines of communication. Repetitive process of trial and error leads to greater motor coordination, but at first with more errors than success. Persistent practice leads to skilled performance, and skilled performance is worthy of earned pride.

The ultimate goal is to have our head crowned with a rich neuropile, i.e., a thick and healthy mat of purposeful neural interconnections. Some brain researchers say that the more complex and interconnected our brain becomes the more intelligent we are. At the very least, a rich and ready neuropile allows for many more possibilities of thought and action.

Finnegan's program has many of the same goals as Kinetic Arts Training. We want every brain to solve problems and be joyous in learning persistence. And his lifetime of work has shown that the act of juggling creates more ambidexterity in the body, and thus more cross-laterality between the right and left brain lobes. Even a small amount of ambidexterity practice helps to balance the brain. Juggling is inherently a bilateral, whole brain skill. A balanced brain is the basis of good physical balance.

> Note: KAT does not ask students to juggle, only to work with the less dominant hand, and little by little bring it to greater functional competency. Of course, a few people want to learn to juggle. They can learn at any age.

The big question is how does the brain do all this? The following facts will not only enlighten but also inspire. They point to our infinite possibilities and offer a guide to our efforts.

As we learned earlier, every time you learn anything new, you forge new neural pathways in your brain. With repetitive use, these pathways become more passable and familiar. Learning is now easier and faster, because you can more easily communicate from one brain location to another. You are now more organized. You started with your genetic blueprint but the rest was your doing. All formal and informal schooling is bent on brain organization, or at least it should be. And we are "sentenced" to brain-bettering-school for life.

I digress a moment to make a meaningful comparison between the brain and the heart. They are very different, of course, but they are also quite similar. Both continually work for our survival and never ask for over-time pay. They do it because they are loyal, even in the face of abuse. Your lifestyle decisions directly affect their function. When your lifestyle decisions are in line with biological realities, your heart and brain serve you well.

Did you know that, in an average lifetime, the heart beats two-and-a-half billion times? When was the last time you thanked your heart? Did you know that if your blood vessels were all laid end to end, they would go around the earth two-and-a-half times? We have been given a magnificent bio-structure but we rarely thank it with the heartfelt gratitude it deserves. Our genuine appreciation for this gift is best expressed when we do everything possible to allow ourselves to function as we were designed.

The heart is magnificent, but the brain is galactic. The pulse of the brain is thought. We can think in as many different ways as there are stars. When we understand our fundamental capabilities, we can achieve the coveted goal of long-lasting, exuberant mental and physical health.

The brain is ready to learn, that is its function. In the last 20 years, we have learned more about the brain than we have learned since the dawn of history. We don't know everything about the brain yet, but we do know a lot. Here are some facts that will let you know what your brain is made of.

Some Brain Facts

A recent book, *The Three-Pound Universe*, by Judith Hooper and Dick Teresi, tell us that we are exceptional beings and that it's our brain that makes us so. It has been said that our three-pound brain is more complicated than the entire universe. Plainly, the human brain is much more amazing than we ever thought. In a 150-pound person, the brain comprises only two percent of the body weight, yet it requires 20 percent of the body's oxygen production. The brain is obviously a vital organ or it would not require and get all this attention. Evidently, importance comes in small packages.

In the 1960s, I read *An Outline of Man's Knowledge of the Modern World* (Bryson Lyman, editor). One paragraph hit me like a ton of bricks:

> *There are over ten billion neurons in the human brain, and each of the larger ones has an average of more than ten thousand connections – synapses – from other neurons! The possible number of network patterns that could be formed, or paths that nerve impulses might travel, is far greater than the total number of particles in the Universe.*

By 1965, scientists had learned enough about the brain to calculate that it contained 30 billion neurons instead of the 10 billions previously thought. That estimate is now very much out of date. In the 1990s we found that, not only is our universe much larger and more complicated than we thought but so is the brain.

In a recent book, *A User's Guide to the Brain: Perception, Attention and the Four Theaters of the Brain,* John J. Ratey, MD, informs us there are 100 billion neurons in the brain. Those 100 billion neurons are the framework for a possible 40 quadrillion connections. Whatever the exact number, it is certain that the brain is fabulous beyond belief. Here are some reasons why.

Through out history, mankind has wondered about our biology. Here is a wonderful fact that can now be stated in numbers. Each brain neuron requires immense amounts of oxygen and nourishment. To accomplish this task 10 glial cells (*glial* means glue) surround each neuron. They are called astrocytes because of their star shape. They provide support and nutrition, and help to establish the blood/brain barrier that keeps unwanted molecules away from brain cells. Brain neurons, along with the astrocytes, add up to at least a trillion cells in the brain. (And this is not counting the cells that make up the veins and arteries, along with the blood they carry).

A Little History

One hundred years ago, the Spanish anatomist Santiago Cajal discovered the brain neuron. He soon realized that the number of brain interconnections and pathways was astronomical. Scientists feel confident in speculating that the number of usable pathways in the brain correlates to levels of intelligence.

Diamond, a creative Psychologist, has taught at The University of California at Berkley for more than 30 years. In the 1960s, Dr. Marion Diamond discovered that rats placed in rich environments were healthier and learned faster than rats living in poor environments. A rich environment, for a rat, meant having bright, spacious cages full of challenging activities and rat toys. When she measured these animals' brains, they weighed more, and had more complex matted neuropiles than those brains of the rats raised in poor environments. Rats raised in rich environments demonstrated higher levels of learning ability. Also, their ability to shunt oxygen to those places in the brain where it was needed was more efficient. The animals brought up in poor environments were just the opposite. They were dull and sickly, and low in tested intelligence. Recently, brain imaging has demonstrated that this phenomenon is true of humans as well: our brains thrive in rich environments. KAT has been designed with these facts in mind. It provides a rich environment full of opportunities for motor learning and brain stimulation.

Dr. Diamond understands that when studying the brain, it is essential to keep in mind that development and aging are on a continuum. For example, from the moment you are born, you begin to age. Your brain does not simply "develop" in the first part of your life and "age" in the last part of your life. While your brain was forming in embryo, it was developing about 50,000 nerve cells per second. Think of that explosive development: *50,000 cells per second.* But by the time of birth, you had already lost at least 50 percent of those cells. Many of us are concerned about losing nerve cells toward the end of our life cycle when, in reality, we lost a lot of nerve cells before entering the world.

Dr. Diamond writes: "If I can now introduce a relevant experience when teaching in Africa in 1988, my husband, Dr. Arnold Scheibel, and I found that in Nairobi, Kenya, pregnant women would not eat protein because it meant they would have to deliver a large baby. It was much easier, in their view, to reduce their protein intake as a way of assuring a smaller baby and an easier delivery. My immediate question, as you might have guessed, was: 'what effect does this reduced protein intake have on the infant brain?' That became the subject of a series of experiments in my laboratory as soon as we returned. One of my graduate students, Arianna Carughi, fed half the pregnant rats a normal, high-protein diet and the other half a low-protein diet. When the babies were born, first of all, the body weight of babies, whose mothers were fed the reduced-protein diet, was found to be 50 percent less than those babies whose mothers had been given a normal protein diet. And the brains? The dendrites in baby rats whose mothers had reduced protein did not develop fully. When we placed the protein-deprived babies in enriched living conditions with lots of objects to explore, the dendrites did not increase significantly, as they did in babies whose mothers had a normal protein diet and enriched living conditions. It was clear that a protein-rich diet is vital to grow healthy nerve cells that can respond positively to enriched living conditions.

Dr. Diamond mentions the importance of good infant nutrition. Let me add that our brain demands a well balanced diet all our lives. Feed it well.

The nervous system changes to accommodate what it senses as a challenge to the organism. When an older person's independence is negatively challenged by age-related neurological declines, the nervous system can restructure itself to restrain that dogged, age-related retreat. Just to stay even with yesterday's level of functioning requires added attention, practice, and diligence. Poetically, I suggest that growing older is an Olympic event where our competitors are the facts of biology.

We easily accept the fact that children learn a phenomenal amount every day. But how is it possible for an old dog to learn new tricks? The truth is that regardless of age, we all can continue to learn. Our learning mechanism is always in the "on" position so we can move up to higher levels of knowledge and skills. Motor learning stimulates an extraordinary reciprocity between the body and brain. Simply put, as the body tries something new the brain is being changed. Each time a skill is practiced, the brain changes and renders learning more permanent.

In recent years we have come to understand that the brain is exceedingly malleable. Neuroscientists have given the term *neuroplasticity* to this characteristic. Connections between brain cells can grow by as much as 25 percent in rich environments. Also, a recent discovery informs us that new nerve cells are continually being created even in elderly persons. Fred Gage was the researcher who discovered this fact. Thanks, Fred!

Intention, Learning, and Skilled Behavior

Mankind has been creatively learning new ways for a very long time. Forty thousand years ago, even a small error could kill you and your entire clan. The possibility of death gets people's attention. Our ancestors learned fast and passed on their survival skills to the next generation. Without these skills, we would not have survived as a species.

Modern society is just as stringent in its demands for adjustment. Inspiring ideas, stimulating objects and intriguing activities help the brain grow to meet life's challenges. In fact, the brain is designed to adjust to environmental changes. The compensatory mechanism of self-awareness allows us to be critical of our errors and learn from them. The intention to be self-critical heightens the analysis of our trial-and-error process. Intention joins with attentiveness to promote adjustment. Over time, we learn new skills, procedures, protocols, practices, and talents. These proficiencies not only keep us alive, but also increase our innate awareness.

It must be remembered that motor actions begin with the intention to develop a performable skill. Even getting up from a chair begins with the intention to do so. A baby's innate drives express themselves as intentions. Later, intention is made purposeful by millions of trials and errors. Errors are good, as long as they are examined attentively, self-critically, and with the goal of future error-free performance. Repeated rehearsal leads to better performance. When there is a oneness of purpose in goal achievement, success is more assured.

There are always spin-offs from learning anything. For example, when your body learns better balance, you may become more daring, perhaps dancing when you have not danced in years, or safely trying what you were afraid to try before. Small successes are significant for the body, mind and soul. Why? Because you did it on your own.

The thrust of Karla Hannaford's book *Smart Moves*, is embedded in its subtitle, *Why Learning Is Not All in Your Head.* Hannaford says that the brain guides the body, but at the same time, the brain learns to be a better guide by listening to the body. The body is wired to do the brain's bidding, and at the same time, the brain is wired to respond to the body's needs and limitations. The outcome of our intention is shown when we exhibit more skill, more grace, smoother action, a calmer performance, and most of all, a greater capability to learn without end.

Structurally, the brain is extremely complicated. This book is not the place for a detailed discussion of anatomy, except one most pertinent fact. Near the top of the brain, there are two thin, adjacent slices of brain tissue. The function of one is language; the function of the other is motor control. Because these two are next-door neighbors, they can quickly and easily communicate. This is one reason why we "talk" so effectively with our hands. Brain imaging shows that the language portion of the brain is active when a deaf person uses their hands and fingers to sign.

This language-motor connection is discussed by Mel Levine in his book: *All Kinds of Minds,* He states, "Fascinating dialogues occur between language and gross motor functions; during the early stages of gross motor development skill, kids use verbal self-coaching. They actually talk their way through an emerging skill." This connection does not stop with childhood. We all benefit by talking out loud to ourselves as we move through the learning process. The connection between language and motor skill development should not seem strange. After all, the body parts that produce language are nerve-muscles driven.

Here is an anecdote about learning language. My wife and I had an extended stay in Europe. We only knew English. We met many people who knew two and even three languages. We also met three persons who were obviously not functioning well; in fact, they were well below average in intelligence. But in spite of low overall intelligence, they each spoke three languages. The point? What did that make us with only one language? We learned fast.

The following may sound facetious but listen to its serious side. I heard a man call his dog in German. The dog understood and obeyed. I thought at the time, even the dog is smarter than me. However, the point is I had only been exposed to English and the dog only to German. We can do and understand only what we have practiced and learned. Just as with a foreign language, balance is a skill to be practiced. Watch a baby learn to walk. Now that's persistent practice. And we all did it. Till our last moments of life, we can and need to learn. Perennial and persistent practice is required for a lifetime.

The way to encourage someone's brain and body toward better balance is to create a series of safe mind/motor "emergencies" which the person must work through. More gently, these "emergencies" are called challenges. Learning a new language especially when immersed in that country is a good example of such a challenge. If these challenges are met, the result is a higher-level skill performance. Learning is made possible by the development, over time, of fundamental changes in brain/body nerve patterning. These emerging patterns or connections are then immediately used as templates, or as stepping-stones, toward the next level of learning. In the case of KAT, the proof of the learning is demonstrated in more stable physical balance.

This has been stated before in one of the best-know principles of architecture: "*Form follows function, function follows form.*" Function (performance), and form (structure) are also applicable to us as humans, although human beings are more complicated than any inanimate building. The brain has the power to choose those bits of learning that are good and unlearn the old stuff. Learning new motor patterns, via trial and error, influences the growth of new connective structures in the brain so that it has better control over the body's performance. This is why our ability to learn can get better and better.

Bugental's seven steps are here repeated for emphasis. To get thing done you must first have an *intention,* which grows into *a wish*, then *a want*, progressing to *desire,* then to *will, action, actualization* and if enough power is generated by action, an *interaction* follows. At this point, the job is completed. Omit any one of these steps and the original intention remains fragmentary.

Five Characteristics of a Healthy Human Brain

In the 1980s, Leslie Hart stated that there were five characteristics of a healthy brain. His formulation is still up to date.

1. The brain is *aggressive*. It is built to pursue learning.
2. The brain is *gated* and *gaited.* It can choose which neural cell gate to open and close. Decisions and choice are the outcomes. Also, the brain has an accelerator and brake. It can gallop, trot, canter, or walk or it can lie down on the trail of life.
3. The brain loves to *talk*. We are designed to represent the world with words i.e., symbols. Language is our special way of manipulating the world and learning about it through thought and expression of thought.
4. The brain abhors a *threat* and shuts down under condition of stress, domination, codependence, or fear.
5. The brain is a *trial-and-error* mechanism. The brain is rewarded by a successful trial,

while error teaches it what not to do. Trial and error form a partnership to generate progressively more accurate brain pathways that ultimately turn our learning into thoughts, memories, and behaviors.

Commit Hart's five points to memory. Then, at any time, you can compare your present behavior to Hart's five-point standard for a healthy brain. An example of the first point. It is sometimes right to be aggressive. But it is sometimes, under other conditions, just as right to be passive. You must decide. When you keep these five points in your mind and observe your own behavior and that of others, you are watching brains work out their trial-and-error experiments in real time.

Learning to play a musical instrument is a good example of the trial-and-error process. At the beginning, a novice musician makes many mistakes. Many fewer mistakes are made when the skill has been finely tuned. One anatomical reason for this is that accomplished musicians have practiced long hours to make sure it all happens right. Practice induces the brain to rewire itself to remember the right way to play. From then on, the new wiring acts a guide in future performances.

Here is an amazing finding. When a young person begins learning to play a stringed instrument, his or her left hand must learn very delicate and intricate fingering. When researchers performed brain scans on long-time string players, they found that the area of the brain responsible for the left hand and fingers was significantly larger than that same area in the non-musicians. That area was also more thickly matted with neural pathways. These musicians had started learning when they were young, when their brains were more supple and amenable to creating new pathways. However, it is reassuring to know that a healthy older brain can still restructure itself; learning can occur till the day of death.

The brain and body both depend on the same vascular and nervous system for life and function. Please consider this. The nervous system begins to lose function by about 30 years of age. The loss is not great till around mid life. Many people become unfit at this age and begin to lose neural function at about two percent a year. Contrast this with a person who remains fit into old age. This person's nervous system depreciates only about half a percent a year. And all because of sensible attention to a prudent diet and judicious exercise. This fitness factor is demonstrated in the person's vigor and quality of life.

It does, however, take a lot of problem solving to stay fit and mentally alert in an older body. Problem solving is also a practiced skill, and is nowhere better practiced than in learning motor skills. The tools chapter offers many such practices.

Eight Components of Intelligence

Howard Gardner's book, *Intelligence Reframed: Multiple Intelligences for the 21st Century*, has caused a fundamental shift in our understanding of intelligence. He states there is not just one but at least eight intelligences. He has identified: *Spatial, Intrapersonal, Interpersonal, Musical, Mathematical*, Bodily-kinesthetic, Linguistic and Existential. Only the first seven are considered practical for our balance practice. Existential is here omitted. The Mnemonic code for these seven is easily remembered. It is S I I M M B E L, pronounced symbol.

Gardner is a psychologist at Cornell University. He emphasizes that each person has all eight intelligences, although usually one or two act as a core to the others. However, for a person to be well rounded, all eight need to be practiced separately and then in different combinations.

Gardner's findings reinforce Kinetic Arts Training efforts to create specific exercises and activities that require more than one intelligence category to be practiced at the same time. The goal is to get these 'separate' intelligences to interact, which results in synergetic enhancement. In the Knowledge Tools section, you will see how many of the tools provide this synergy. (I have Gardner's personal permission to say that he has verified the above premise. Our visit was indeed a privilege.)

Of course, genetics plays a part in the quality of an individual's intelligence, but so does learning. When you know what these are intelligences are, you can work toward their development.

Each of these seven intelligences has its own primary control mechanisms in the brain. Practice is the catalyst for the process of interconnection. A connected brain is a balanced brain.

All of Gardner's intelligence categories are relevant to a balanced life. However, their interaction and effectiveness is different in all of us. It is best to practice in all areas. Remember that growth of one area has influence on all the others.

Neural Integration (Synergy)

Buckminster Fuller brought the concept of synergy into popular use with his 1954 invention of the geodesic dome. Fuller says that the behavior of a whole system is unpredictable from the behavior of its parts taken separately. Fuller suggests synergistic outcomes are always a surprise. A medical definition simply tells us that synergy occurs when parts work cooperatively together. Cooperative interaction produces significantly more output than the sum total of the parts working separately.

Here is an example from the Wisconsin fair. A team of very large Belgian draft horses lunged forward at precisely the same time, moving a phenomenal load. The same principle of unity is true for us. When all the components of the nervous system work for the good of the whole, we can say we really have it together. That togetherness is orchestrated by a brain and a body working synergistically as one.

Please allow me to drive home the point. The human body is composed of approximately 30 trillion cells. All 30 trillion cells work cooperatively to demonstrate this magnificent unity. Life seems to be a synergetic outcome of our vast biological cellular diversity, displayed by the variety in organs, and systems. Just as synergy is integral to our body and brain, it is also at work in the neural integration produced by KAT practice. Here are three lines stated before. They say a lot.

When I point my mind, it is this that I find.
I get what I earn when I earn what I learn,
that my body and mind, are always entwined.

Three Avenues of Brain Integration

We conceive of the world through our uniquely interconnected neural network. Brain Gym offers a simplified, three avenue approach to understanding brain integration. Brain Gym is a widely used series of exercises designed to calm and integrate the nervous system. Its formulation offers clues to what exercises may be most helpful. All three avenues contribute to solid balance. Each requires continual strengthening, as do their interactions. The three brain dimensional avenues are:

left-to-right reciprocal communication,
back-to-front focus; and
top-to-bottom centering.

Left-to-Right Reciprocal Brain Lobe Communication

Cross-brain lobe communication is the back-and-forth interaction between the two brain lobes. The term cross-lateral is also used for this linkage. An example will make it practical. Left-to-Right Brain Lobe Communication occurs when an object is passed or tossed from one hand to the other. Ambidextrous persons seem to be first-rate in this ability. But non-ambidextrous people can also benefit greatly from practicing cross lateral activities. Some examples are jugglers, baseball switch-hitters, and pianists. And there are many simpler exercises to get started. All coordination between both hands opens up these brain lines of communication.

A famous historical example of ambidexterity was Leonardo da Vinci. One of his personal habits was continually refining his ambidexterity. He must have intuitively known that it was good for his ability to think. Leonardo was a juggler, a musician, and a painter, and much more. The stories about his painting with either hand are unparalleled. When he was tired of painting with one hand, he just switched to the other. He really did use his brain more efficiently than the average person. His works and life attest to the superior training of his brain.

> Note: Leonardo was a juggler, which gives me hope. At my age, not really much hope . . . but 500-year-old hope is better than nothing.

Back-to-Front Reciprocal Brain Focus

Our eyes, located at the front of the head, receive visual information, which is sent to receptor neurons in the back of the brain for interpretation. Good communication between the front and the back is vital. Vision is responsible for 30 to 40 percent of balance. But *sight* may also be understood as insight, imagination, and intuition. Our brain can make pictures that are not mere reproductions of things in the world. Imagination and insight are part of 'seeing' our goals as if they are already reached.

Accurate vision, as well as good control of your eyes, requires practice. Later I will talk about attention-switching exercises that help the eyes remain serviceable. Knowing where to look is a practiced skill, as is control of the neck muscles. I love the line that goes, "*When you learn where to look in life, you will become better looking.*" Good-looking people never bump into others who may not be looking as good as you.

Top-to-Bottom Reciprocal Brain Centering

Our thinking centers are on the top of the brain while the motor centers are at the base of the brain. Messages, (decisions), are initiated from the top and travel all the way down the spine to the legs and then into our feet. That remarkable nerve communication keeps us balanced. Upright balance is learned at a very young age. But balance can be affected by advancing age, disease, disuse, and injury, all of which can intensify neurological decline. Under these conditions, we must relearn how best to use our diminishing resources to keep ourselves safe from falls. Part of safe balance may be rehabilitation of certain parts of the nervous system. Some of the ways that you can make the most of the rest of your life are surgery, physical therapy, stopping bad habits, practicing new way of locomotion, and bettering your life style. Any way you look at it, balance is stability and independence. One nicely metered and very serious statement is:

When you place your feet in the right place,
at the right time, all the time,
you will never fall.

The trick to be ready all the right time, and all the time, so imbalance recovery abilities are ready when needed. KAT exercises and activities are designed to this end. (See the last chapter on Tools.)

Automaticity

Have you ever wondered how you can walk and talk at the same time, and do both without contemplating each step or word? One word for this is *automaticity.* Automaticity is defined as the ability of the body to perform a skilled movement without volitional attention. This ability takes time and effort. Automaticity of a motor skill requires repeated trial and error, willed persistence, and sometimes the patience of Job.

The observable outcome of this process is smooth and confident motor action. Complicated bio-systems could never do all they do without much of their daily movement being automatic. Here is an example of automaticity in action. In the 1950s, I worked in an Army hospital. I scheduled at least 10 minutes of practice a day to learn to juggle with my eyes closed. Practicing with eyes closed made my somatosensory system more capable as it took over the responsibility of the eyes. After a year of practice, I could "see" the balls with my mind's eye, through my hands. My tosses and catches have become so automatically accurate that the balls land where they can be caught. And if I bobble a ball and/or toss it a bit off course, I instantly adjust the other hand to make up for the mistake. All highly skilled movements come from long, concentrative practice. Also, I need to mention that after more than 55 year since learning the skill, I can still juggle blind. A motor skill, once learned, has staying power. All of us have generated automatic skills such as running or playing a musical instrument. You have the power to learn new ones.

The other side of this is that there are some things that need to be unlearned as we become older, diseased or injured. Unlearning is best accomplished by replacing the old pattern with a better, more useable skill. Same process, practice till it becomes automatic.

A psychologist friend, who was intrigued by my blind juggling, hooked me to his neuro-feedback computer. His program breaks down EEG patterns into the brain's beta, alpha and theta waves. The screen showed that my brain was 100% in beta as I juggled three balls with my eyes open. Beta is the active, wide-awake brain state. The instant I closed my eyes, still juggling three balls, my brain switched from beta to alpha. Alpha is the dream state, that transitional state between waking and sleeping. The alpha state is very introspective and is required for deep concentration. His interpretation was that my practice had made my brain capable of almost instantaneous adjustment to the demands of blind juggling.

But, you may say, that story is nothing special; *all* learning requires concentration. I agree. High levels of concentration and focus are latent in all of us. Even injured brains have the power to make a motor skill automatic. When new learning is desired, practice makes it automatic.

In the process, the skill becomes recognizably smoother because the brain has now restructured the template from long practice. How about that! Thank you, brain, for complying with my desires. And my brain might reply, *"but master, didn't you know that's my duty"*

The body/mind unit is an instrument that requires continual reanalysis, reworking and rerouting. Are you walking in the most efficient manner? Are you lifting things so you don't injure your back? Are you living in line with the rules of human physiology? If not, you can change. Our will has the power to change our lifestyle.

Attention

Attention just may be the most important concept related to optimum brain functioning. I sincerely hope I can do justice to this all-encompassing human faculty.

I am not a chess player but one of my heroes is Bobby Fischer, a world chess champion. He demonstrated enormous attention in his game. How did he do it? A partial answer is that he knew that being physically fit was a part of mental focus. He kept himself in top shape. Even during his matches, he would get up between chess moves and keep his body limber, which helped his mind retain its focus.

In this same vein, I told my University students that I resented it when they smoked. I stated, "Did you know that smoking reduces your oxygen uptake by 10 percent? That means that you smokers are 10 percent less able than you could be. And you do it by choice. If someone said to you, 'You're not all there,' they'd be right." Attention detractors, of any sort, must be eliminated.

Crossword puzzles and the game of bridge are often thought of as good brain-food. I would agree that they demand concentration, a wide store of knowledge and disciplined thinking. These two great games stimulate the brain well, but most bridge players have not listened to Bobby Fischer.

If people can get out of bed to play bridge, they can get up from the their bridge game more often, walk around the table, and start playing again with their brains and bodies refreshed. An ample blood supply to the brain is vital for high attention levels. Also, movement and stretching relieve physical and mental stress. Physical activity increases oxygen to the brain

and the brain does require oxygen in large quantities. The more I think of Bobby Fischer, the more of a health model he becomes.
The word 'attention' is worth checking out in the Oxford English Dictionary. It defines attention as: *The action, fact, or state of attending or giving heed: earnest direction of the mind, consideration or regard.* But attention is more than this; it has many connotations. The following is a list of 17 synonyms. These 17 words will broaden your view of attention.

Seventeen Synonyms for Attention

Alert	Considerate	On guard
Analyze	Earnestness	On the ball
Attentive	Focus	Thoughtful
Awareness	Heedful	Vigilance
Concentration	Intent	Wakefulness
Consciousness	Mindfulness	

Attention may be categorized in three ways:

Selective – concentrative, focused, conscious, laser-like, direct, hard focus
Divided – alternating, peripheral, concurrent, soft focus
Mixed – all the above.

A healthy brain "chooses" to use one of the above categories depending on situational demands. Focused attention links us to our consciousness.

In the field of philosophy, attention is defined as that state of being characterized by sensation, emotion, thought. Now let's add Webster's definition: *Consciousness is the awareness of something within oneself; also the state or fact of being conscious in regard to some thing.* Webster rounds out his definition with: *The totality of the conscious states: a mind in a normal conscious state of life.*

That last line is really something. Consciousness is a normal state of mind, and yet the book, *Waking Up*, by Charles Tart, tells us that we are 'asleep at the switch' much of the time. Yet, we know that consciousness is the semantic brother to Attention. This family's motto has to be:

Conscious attention makes life worth living.

A fully conscious, actively attentive person is a wide-awake, on-the-money, and with-it kind of person. Solving motor problems is an especially good method for keeping our attention intact. Solving motor problems demands a high level of conscious awareness of both the inside and the outside the body. An object cannot be tossed hand-to-hand without simultaneous internal and external awareness. Thus, we must remind ourselves to consciously monitor our thoughts, feelings, and functions as we perceive and manipulate the outside world. Again, the goal is to maintain and even enhance our brain's ability to connect inside and outside realms. The neurological term for this is *concurrency*, doing more than one thing at a time. Here I specifically applied the term to attending to the inside and the outside world at the same time. Later you will find more detail on concurrency, and the value of practicing doing more than one thing at a time.

Psychologists have long studied the learning process. As of late, psychology has placed awareness and consciousness side by side with learning as a legitimate area for study. The fields of neurology, anatomy and psychology have joined forces to study brain functioning under varied conditions, a specialty known as neuroscience. At the base of all learning is the high-level awareness of both the outside world and those neurological memory and learning processes within. Healthy levels of alertness help us cope with the frustrations of life and learning. Attention focuses thought and drives us to what we want to achieve. The ability to attend can be enhanced.

There is another side of attention. It is the power of ignoring whatever is not part of our intentional thought focus. The ability to ignore distractions is as much a skill as the ability to focus. Children and adults with attention deficit disorder fail to ignore things not central to their learning purpose. They are deluged by too much competing information. Normalcy requires a balance between ignoring and direct focus. (The tools chapter has some tips on how to practice this skill.)

As teachers and parents remind their children, I remind you to "*pay* attention." The emphasis is on the word *pay.* Attention is paid for with desire, purpose, intention, will and energy. The conduit for paying attention is via sensation, emotion, and thought. You, in the broadest sense, are worth paying attention to. Your health is your lifeline to a worthwhile future. We say, take care of yourself. The emphasis in on *your self.* No one wants your health as much as you. When you pay attention to improving yourself, you then have the power to invest attention in other pursuits. It's a nice thing to do.

In many ways, we humans are given the ability to lift ourselves up by our own bootstraps. For example, willpower underlies all conscious action and thought. There are three foundational forces of will. It all starts with *attention.* Attention gives rise to *intention*, intention give direction to *volition*, and volition adds direction and power to *will.* These four human traits must also be kept in top shape. When not used, they too decline in ability and power. Willpower is augmented by thinking and doing. Full consciousness is the active exercise that requires all four, *attention, intention, volition, and will.*

When I point my mind, it is this that I find.
I get what I earn when I earn what I learn,
that my body and mind, are always entwined.

Balance Systems

Three Balance Control Systems

Each of these three systems relays differing kinds of balance information to the brain. The *somatosensory* system contains billions of skin, muscle and joint sensors, which inform the brain about temperature, pressure and movement. It informs us of any muscle contractions and/or muscle elasticity, as well as telling us the angle at which our joints are positioned at any one time.

The *visual* system is composed of the eyes. Our eyes view the world and provide information about our spatial orientation and the nature of our immediate environment, a function that keeps us safely avoiding potholes.

The *vestibular system* (the inner ear) tells us when our head is off center. More specifically, it registers changes in gravitational, linear, and angular accelerations of the head in space. The body depends on the vestibular system completely when vision and the somatosensory system are disabled.

Coordinated feedback and feed-forward among these three systems is essential for solid balance.

I like to think of these three neurological systems as three musical instruments. Each of the three performs a different function in the physical balance "orchestra." Of course, the acknowledged conductor is the brain itself. The three instruments, i.e., the three balance systems are briefly described below.

The Somatosensory System

The somatosensory system makes a unique contribution to our balance. (Soma = body. Sensory = awareness of our inside and outside worlds.) Sensory *afferent* nerves are embedded in every muscle fiber, in all joints and in all the surfaces of the body. Their job is to tell us where we are in space relative to the floor, to locate our center of gravity, and indicate where our body parts are relative to one another. Neuroanatomists classify these nerve fibers as *tactile*, *deep pressure*, *joint receptor*, and *proprioceptor* nerves. With the information received from the *afferent* nerves, the *efferent* sends control impulses to the muscles.

Tactile Nerves - The sense of touch is located all over the body. Especially rich in tactile nerves are the soles of the feet, the palms of the hands, and the mouth, lips and tongue. All of these body parts are richly endowed with nerves because each has a distinct task in keeping us productive and safe. For example, those masses of tactile nerves on the soles of our feet let us know when we are rocking back on our heels or up on our toes. Tactile nerves also sense temperature, pressure, and pain.

Deep Pressure Nerves - There are sensing nerves deep inside every muscle. They inform us whether a muscle is relaxed or contracted. Also, these sensors tell us when a muscle is being stretched beyond its safe range of motion.

Joint receptors - These sensory nerves inform the brain at what angle the joint is bent and when the joint is being forced beyond its mechanical limits. Also, these joint receptors tell us the relative position of each joint in relation to adjacent limbs and the rest of the body. Joint receptors help us know where we are in space.

Propreoceptors - These sensors are also in every muscle fiber. They tell the brain where in space a muscle is in relation to adjacent muscles. They also inform the brain if muscles are being stretched beyond their safe limits.

The somatosensory system provides a most important defense against postural imbalance. It works in conjunction with vision and the inner ear.

The Vision System

Vision informs us of our relationship to the environment. The ability to see at a distance allows us to avoid potholes and other pitfalls, and interact with the environment in a safe and meaningful manner. Information gathered at a distance gives us time to think and decide how to navigate the world safely. It is true that blind people ambulate quite well. The reason? They are kept reasonably balanced by the exceptionally well-practiced components of the somatosensory and vestibular systems. However, for those who are sighted, vision enables smoother and more graceful movement. Vision is even more important when the supporting surface is unstable. When our eyes and somatosensory systems work together, they do almost the entire job of balancing for us.

The Vestibular System (The Inner Ear)

The third balance system is the vestibular system, which senses angular and/or linear acceleration of the head as it moves in space, as well as the force of gravity.
For example, when we quickly turn our head from side to side, or when we are quickly yanked up or down on an elevator or in an airplane, our inner ear senses these motions. The three semicircular canals in the inner ear are structurally designed to perform these sensory tasks. This ability is vital for the body's performance of complex, coordinated movements. The vestibular system is the system least used for normal activities but when the somatosensory and/or visual systems are disrupted, the vestibular system plays a larger role in our balance.

Our balance is solid when all three systems are healthy. When they optimally interact, we do fine. However, if one or the other has trouble sending correct information to the brain, we are in trouble. If two of the three systems are viable, we will remain passably balanced. But, of course, having all three in good working order is best. A trip or stumble demands fast, competent, and accurate reactions from all systems. These three systems are in place for a good reason. Each has a special function that assures good balance.

The American College of Sports Medicine as well as Richard Restak suggests that when you enhance any one part of the body system, you enhance all other parts of the body at the same time. This is not only true of the physical but is also true of the mental, social, emotional, and spiritual parts of us. Who said the body was less important than the brain? They scratch each other's back. When we lack neural integration, we lack balance.

The three main balance systems, along with all chemical, morphological and functional systems must communicate optimally to produce vigorous health and good balance. Each and every cell in the body has the power to detract from or contribute to our balance. This is why good overall body conditioning and good nutrition is a health requirement.

Other Balance Influences

Environmental factors can affect our sense of balance. A railing on the stairs can insure your safety. Icy roads can cause falls. We can consciously decide to install a railing and avoid or adjust appropriately to ice. Environmental factors can add or detract from safe balance. Thus, there is great importance to design our environment as safe as possible, as well as to maximize all the functions of all three neurological balance systems.

Perception

Our perception is oft times attracted to non-safety concern. More frankly, we don't look where we're going. But there is hope. Perception devoted to safety can be enhanced. There are three ways. First, realistically know your environment, second, know your fitness level and balance skill capacity, and third, prepare for neurological decline by putting up railings, using a cane, etc. More perception and attention skills are detailed in the next two chapters.

Here's an example of a perception failure. A friend of mine was much too active before his stitches fully healed. He became infected and paid the price. Right perception would have told him what he could not healthfully do, and then open up the search for what he could and should do.

Perception is more than visual. The eyes are connected to the brain's decision centers that control where we look and what we think about what we see. Simply, seeing a stumbling block is not enough; we must decide to avoid it. Learning where to look will help you remain the good looker you are.

Here is another way to appreciate the concept of *to look*. Your body is organized so that when your eyes look left, your head following the eyes, and your shoulders, hips, and feet soon follow. Where you go has to do with where you look.

T*o look* has another meaning. It occurs when you delve into the details of some new and interesting idea. Interesting ideas activate the mind and body. This activation is felt as life's vitality. Vitality is energy, which is required to remain balanced in the face of any debilitating condition. We humans are capable of looking on both sides of a question, considering many possible decision paths, and entertaining matters of personal health in relation to public health. This capability allows others to see us in the light of our knowledge, our quality, and our zest for learning and sharing. Good friends always see each other as interesting and good-looking because they dig under the surface for a really good look.

In a sense, high interest in life pays health dividends. High interest in ideas and learning influences how we look at ourselves, how we know ourselves, and what we do about our faults and blemishes. And it all started with a good perceptive look.

Outcomes of Right Looking

To see the world in a grain of sand
And a heaven in a wild flower;
Hold infinity in the palm of your hand
And eternity in an hour.
Blake

Note: Blake's attitude is to be emulated. His metaphors are powerful.

Excellent perception is highlighted by three words: *stop*, *look*, and *listen*. Adherence to these three words has prevented many a fall. The poet William Blake also knows something about perception.

Right looking can be demonstrated when:

Your *wisdom* becomes apparent. Your *passion* becomes infectious.
Your *intelligence* becomes uplifting. Your *calmness* becomes rehabilitating.
Your *helpfulness* becomes contagious. Your *sharing* becomes liberating.
Your *empathy* becomes regenerative. Your *listening* becomes supportive.
Your *joy* becomes invigorating. And your *self* becomes your own best friend.

Blake reflects the "here and now" philosophy. His view is paraphrased as alertness of the moment. Perception of this quality blocks out the past and the future, and allows great concentration on the present. You have the power to purposefully assign your personal presence to right now. In this state of mind, your view is as focused as the brilliant sun streaming through a pinhole on a black sheet of paper. Blake is suggesting that the present is the only time that is real. The past is past and the future is not yet here. To be in the here and now means that you are alert in your body and mind, within each moment of time. And that's exactly what perennial balance requires.

Bad Habits

Bad habits detract from balance. They are yesterday's decisions gone sour. An example of an unhealthy habit is thinking that we are as good as we ever were and as we will ever be. The truth is, we all have the potential to change for the better . . . or worse.

Here's an example. The findings of medical researchers now encourage heart-attack patients to exercise after their surgery, as well as for the rest of their lives. They studied heart-attack patients who followed an exercise routine and lost weight. This group reported feeling and looking better and actually lived longer than the group with no exercise routine. What a life-affirming recommendation for exercise. The other side of this point is a sad state of human affairs. It too often takes a near catastrophe to wake a person up to the value of preventative fitness.

We Are Unique

Knowing we are unique plays a role in our perceptions. Our genetic make-up and our environmental interactions, from birth to the present, make us different from any other person. Also, our experiences and our interpretations of those experiences are particularly unique to us. No wonder we look at things differently from other people. Knowing we are unique allows us to know that everyone else is unique. Empathy for another point of view is extraordinarily healthy.

Fear and Denial

Our perceptions can easily be altered by our physical condition and/or state of mind. Fear, for instance, exacerbates falls. Fear freezes muscle actions and reactions. When you freeze, you are less able to react to an emergency. Neurology texts strongly make this point. Fear makes you uneasy and anxious, detracting from the attention needed for good balance.

The remedy is to change fear into caution. This switch is more than semantic. Labeling does amazing things to our thinking processes. Caution is not debilitating, rather it liberates energy to find out what needs to be done to eliminate the cause of the fear. Honestly face your fear and latent logic will force caution to emerge.

Also, fear-based biases and prejudices can detract from our optimum functioning. The opposite of fear and denial is acceptance of reality. An honest survey of your situation and yourself will open your eyes and mind to possible corrective actions. There are always more possibilities than seen at first glance. The smart strategy is to prepare for the reality of falling. The Boy Scout motto, 'Be prepared,' can keep you out of a lot of trouble.

Self-Concept

A solid self-concept is born out of learning how to care for oneself. It has to do with a person's understanding of his or her options, developing strategies for gaining greater knowledge, and planning a lifestyle that includes activities for mental and physical fitness.

A good self-concept always sees itself as more than three-dimensional. First, human beings have physical length, width, depth, and thus have biological permanence. The fourth dimension is time, although our earth time is brief. But there's much more. We are physical, mental, emotional, social, moral and spiritual beings; and most likely more. The amazing part is that all these qualities are contained in each and every one of us.

The way you *see* yourself is a health-controlling factor. The trick is to practice being proud of the good things you do. Good acts deserve honest pride. Pride does not precede a fall when pride is justified. Compliments from others feel good but everyone does good things for family and the world without anyone else's knowledge. You are the only one to fully appreciate yourself for your full worth.

There are four types of self-concept. 1. You may realistically know your value, 2. You may put an unrealistically high value on yourself, i.e., if you have an inflated ego; or the opposite, 3. You may be slave-like and have no idea of your value, and slavishly do whatever you are told. 4. The best approach is to diligently investigate who in the heck you really are. And if by chance you never come to a satisfactory answer, do not fret, you are not alone. Take consolation in the fact that you definitely *were*, you now *are*, and you *will be* you as long as your loyal heart provides a life-giving pulse. The exciting part comes from the understanding that the journey toward truth is much more fun than fantasy.

A positive self-concept and mental attitude are based on the discipline of perceiving your life and the world in an opportunistic light. The glass of the optimist is always half-full.

Even your choice of words makes a difference to your motivational self. Discipline is a factor of control. It implies "stick-to-itiveness," the ability to concentrate on and dedicate yourself to worthwhile goals. Some people have more of this ability, some have less, while some have none. The discipline of practicing (let's say with a yo-yo) for just a minute a day corresponds to the same discipline used to concentrate on working out a difficult decision. Discipline, concentration, and control are all needed in order to practice satisfactory balance. In fact, as our nervous system declines with age, disease, and injury, these abilities are required more and more. The tool chapter offers many ways to make practice practical.

Entrainment and Concurrency

The decline of our ability to attend corresponds with an age related decline of the nervous system, along with injury, disease, and trauma. Realizing this fact makes the research term *entrainment* important. Entrainment means the body's ability to coordinate attention. The physiology literature suggests that the words *entrainment* and *synchronization* are often used interchangeable.

Concurrency is doing more than one thing at a time. KAT melds entrainment and concurrency to mean the process of attention-guided intentionality, which consciously activates and sustains the learning of new interrelated motor skill behaviors. Simply, this means that better balance is better achieved when attention is marshaled to that end. Good balance, can be said to be an attention exercise.

Human being habitually performs more than one motor skill at a time. However, moving to a higher level of motor skill requires dedicated intentionality and attentionality. This ability is activated and enhanced by repetitive practice, which in turn leads the brain to lay down neural patterns of greater control. Wonderfully, this brings us back full circle to the ability of all muscles and muscle groups to work together. Focused attention takes control of the motor systems which can become more capable than before. Motor learning success is seen in efficient, effortless, purposeful, and coordinated movement.

Gracefulness is a perfect word to describe a well-executed motor skill. The goal is akin to the grace viewed in a harmoniously performed waltz.

Knowledge: A Tool for Balance

Say not, "I have found the truth."
Rather say, " I have found a truth."
Kahlil Gibran

I know what I know, and I never say no
to the new, which tells me to,
go man go!

Obviously, knowledge is life enhancing. I classify knowledge as a tool of balance and health. Even a little knowledge will help to squash ignorance. Good decisions come only in the presence of knowledge. Remember the story of the man walking near a cliff. He literally closed his eyes to the danger and died. He, of course, died from the fall but the real reasons was his decision to blind himself to reality.

All through this book, you will find solid knowledge to guide you toward health and better balance. Right practice, in pursuit of better balance, has much to do with knowing what to do and why to do it. Thus far, this book has provided facts and information, as well as motivational encouragement. This chapter briefly reiterates some of those points and focuses on other ways to know more about how and why of balance practice.

Knowledge as a Tool to Itself

Knowledge is power. Knowledge puts you in the right place at the right time. Knowledge can also put you in the right mental attitude, and promote a solid emotional stance. It fosters the right spiritual posture, and it encourages the right social perspective. Specifically, with regard to balance, knowledge of the sustaining power of physical fitness supports the quality of life that you desire.

Kinetic Arts Training Axiom

It is vital that you become your own balance coach. The KAT balance-enhancing axiom is: *Do what you can, and then a little bit more.* You decide just how much your little bit more is. A lot of littles add up to a *lot.* By the way, the KAT axiom is not only used in the balance class but can be used in the practice of life. Try it.

Three Defenses Against Falls

The *ankles* are the first line of defense. The *hips and step (speedy reaction,)* follow in importance. The three are greatly augmented by conscious attention.

If your ankles' ability to keep your balance fails, the second line of defense is your hip flexibility. And if both of these are pushed beyond their limits of correction, the step comes into play. Ankles need to be strong, hips need to be flexible, and the step needs to be quick. Strength, flexibility and reaction speed can be practiced to better maintain these defensive capabilities.

Ankles Sit in a chair and do ankle circles with one or two feet at a time. Or you can lie in bed with your feet over the end and rotate both ankles. Build up your endurance so you can do a lot of these strengthening circles, but start slowly. Remember that just plain walking is good for keeping the nerve connections from your feet to your brain alive and working. (See the Ice Cream Cone and the Wind Shield Wiper in the next chapter.)

Hips Hip flexibility is your second defense against falls. Bend a lot. Drop things on purpose, so you can pick them up. Become a lint picker-upper. Learn to think of the game of 52 Pick Up as a fun way to stimulate your mind and perfect your balance at the same time. (52 Pick up is detailed in the next section).

Step (speedy leg reactions) Practice quick reactions at the foot, knee and hip. Practice ballet moves at the bar (and I don't refer to the corner tavern). (See Walking Lines and Spots in the next chapter). Speedy reactions are the third line of defense against falls. Keep your interest in life alive and striding forward. Do the same with your body. We dare not forget the *use it or lose it principle.*

Motor Fitness Defined

According to the class notes of my American College of Sports Medicine certification class, the five components of motor fitness are *agility, balance, coordination, power,* and *speed.* Although these five are not mutually exclusive, all five do have their special and unique responsibilities to balance.

Agility Agility is the ability to move quickly and easily, such as being able to rhythmically dance, or type, speak extemporaneously, or safely recover from a stumble.

The three most important words in this definition are *move, quickly,* and *easily.* A fall is caused by loss of balance. To recover, you have to move fast. Fast movements are more easily performed when you can move smoothly and fluidly. But smooth and quick movement does not happen if you have untrained muscles. The colloquial term "Keep loose" means you are ready for anything at any time.

Balance Balance allows you to sustain body stability under normal conditions and make a safe recovery when perturbed. Dynamic balance implies control of movement. The body's state of equilibrium is controlled for a given purpose, such as negotiating stairs, or getting up from a chair or hurrying after a bus.

My childhood understanding of balance was when two kids of equal weight were on a teeter-totter. No action occurs when there's equilibrium. But walking, and even standing depends on dynamic balance. Walking is controlled falling. The brain initiates the impulse to walk, thrusting forward with one foot and catching our selves with the other. Communication between the brain and the body makes this happen. It's strange to think that our brain is as important to locomotion as our legs. Thinking not only makes things happen but better thinking makes better things happen even better.

Coordination Coordination is the organized action of muscles in the performance of complicated movements. This includes dynamic neural cooperation between and among all body parts, functions, and systems, for the purpose of goal-directed survival and optimum consciousness.

The beginning of all learning is the intention to learn. Then, the process of trial and error will progressively forge new brain pathways. The brain is designed to adjust to persistent learning demands. Brain pathways begin as unruly jungle-like trails, but with practice and time, they become super-highways for efficient nerve impulse travel. Bodily coordination depends on a brain with neural pathways programmed for coordinated movement. The next chapter is chock-full full of ways to do just that.

<u>Power</u> Power is the capacity to produce needed muscle force to accomplish a quality life. Maintenance power simply sustains what you have. Greater power is needed when emergencies arise. Many people do not have this extra strength. There is no pill for this safety margin; you have to go after it. Effort is the currency of payment.

Resistance training is the fastest way to gain strength. Progress is heartening, when you start small and work up gradually.

There are many other health benefits from acquiring healthy, strong muscles. One of these is maintaining the immune system. In the November 1999 issue of *Scientific American*, in his essay, "Muscular Again," Glenn Zorpette writes, "Loss of muscle can actually weaken the immune system." He goes on to say, "Also, geriatric health specialists now see muscle loss as underlying many of the injuries to elderly people caused by falling. Thrown off balance, an older person may not have the muscle power necessary to correct posture quickly enough to avoid a nasty fall."

People who have never lifted weights sometimes frown when it is suggested. But if they think about it, they will realize that getting up from a chair or from the floor is weight lifting. In fact a simple and cost-free technique that combines aerobic training for the heart and strength training for the legs and the hips and reducing unneeded fat, is to get down on the floor or sit in a chair and repeatedly get up and down. See the Chair Ups test in the next chapter. The Chair Ups test may be used to measure your progress.

<u>Speed (Reaction Time)</u> Speed equals total distance traveled per unit of time. Here I am talking about neural speed, which promotes timely muscular responses for carrying out purposeful actions and/or avoiding danger.

Speed, or adequate reaction time of all muscles and body functions, contributes to the confidence derived from practice. You don't dare to move fast when you are out of shape, because you may strain something "valuable". But a fit person will respond at whatever speed is required for full and safe function.

The synergy among these five components of motor fitness -- *<u>A</u>gility, <u>B</u>alance, <u>C</u>oordination, <u>P</u>ower*, and *<u>S</u>peed)* is seen in gracefully safe locomotion and confidence in thought and action. These five are easily memorized with the acronym – <u>A</u>. <u>B</u>. <u>C</u>. <u>P</u>. <u>S</u>.

Why memorize the five? Together, these components play a role in balance and health. KAT tools and activities are designed with these five in mind. Each tool is unique yet interrelated. They also can be used as motivational tools to "get with" your practice.

When you know the five by heart, they become consciously accessible. The entire nervous system is enhanced by your efforts to learn new motor patterns. And learning to better balance can be done within your daily routine. The goal is to enhance all you have, and then go on from there to learn more. Why settle for less?

My performance is forever on line,
like the coordination of a meal with fine wine.
I consolidate my ability
with balance and agility.
I have power and speed at the same time.

Body Mass Index (BMI)

Body Mass Index is the ratio of height to weight. With too much weight for height, you are obese. Too little weight is not good either. BMI values apply to both adult men and women, regardless of their age, frame size, or muscle mass. However, they do not apply to athletes or body builders, pregnant or nursing women, frail or elderly persons, or persons under 18. (A special BMI formula is designed for children.) Use BMI information, along with other health indices, to assess your need to change your weight. A BMI of 20 to 24 is healthy, 25 to 29 is overweight, while obesity is equal to or greater than BMI 30.

All you need is your height in inches and your weight in pounds. A responsible person knows body weight is a weighty matter. Try any one of the following web sites for information and calculation. Or for more information consult Google - BMI.

www.consumer.gov/weightloss/bmi.htm or
http://nhlbisupport.com/bmi/ or
www.cdc.gov/nccdphp/dnpa/bmi/index.htm

Body Parts and Systems as KAT Tools

The hands are usually the first body part thought of as a tool. But the shoulders, the back, the legs, and the feet all support the hands in their work. In reality, all body parts have some influence over the balance process.

Fat is a body part. But too much acts as a kind of overabundant, misplaced ballast which makes it more difficult to recover from a stumble. Also too much fat actually creates a substance that enters the blood stream and degrades every organ in the body.

When more body parts or systems purposefully join in a coordinated action, the brain forms new and valuable connections. One vital example is coordination between the upper body and the lower body. When they work together, we can better maintain our center of gravity.

But this is not all. Body parts come together to make up systems. The lungs are a system controlled by brain patterns, which in turn controls nerves, muscles. Oxygen intake is a balance between life and death. For centuries, yoga, tai chi, and meditation have espoused the value of proper breathing. See the next chapter for concurrency exercises, which include respiration. Balance is dependent on every cell in the body to do its job. Let's be dramatic and say it this way:

Each and every cell in the body
can either detract from or contribute to your balance.

All your body's cells are dedicated to your life. If you take care of every cell, you have a quality physiological life. Your health is perched on the fulcrum of choice . . . your choice.

Strength - Flexibility - Aerobics – Balance

The three traditional foci of health gyms have been *strength, flexibility, and aerobics.* These three are the basis of good balance. KAT honors these three, but adds to them the neurology of balance. *On Balance* emphasizes a neurological approach in creating balance enhancement exercises and activities. Thankfully, gyms are beginning to add balance classes to their list of classes. I hope the instructors know their neurology. (See next chapter on physical tools.)

Work from Your Strengths

Kinetic Arts Training strives to enhance all balance processes and systems that are still amenable to improvement. For example, blind people cannot enhance their vision, but they can learn to "see" more with their other senses. Insight is awareness of the outside world interpreted in a realistic manner. When you enhance one sense, all the others are also enhanced. KAT works on and with whatever is available. If you have a reasonably intact central nervous system, you are in the betterment business. Remember the marvelous plasticity of the brain is always there to help . . . and be helped.

One important rule of the Universe says,
when you fall . . . you fall.
But there is another rule that says,
when you avoid a fall, you break rule one.

Ambidexterity

Ambidexterity is generally thought of as the equal use of both hands. But the hands are only part of it. The two lobes of the brain also become more balanced in the process of bilateral practice. When the lesser hand operates in a more coordinated manner, the brain has reprogrammed itself to better coordinate the hand. Ambidexterity is as much in the brain as in the hands.

Open a familiar door for a week with the hand you use least. Your awkwardness will soon be replaced with greater efficacy. Now you're not so one-sided. Ambidexterity was one of Leonardo da Vinci's principles of betterment. He well understood the brain's fantastic capacity to learn. We now know that learning occurs because of the neuroplastic ability of the brain to create new pathways, an ability that can be sharpened at any age. Leonardo amazed onlookers when he painted with either hand. In his own way, he knew his ambidexterity made his brain better. (By the way, we jugglers are proud that Leonardo was one of us.)

As you perform a motor pattern with your best hand, give conscious attention to exactly what you are doing. Thoughtful attention is required for any substantial learning. Then try the same action with your other hand. Make a habit of trying out many daily activities with your lesser-used hand.

Here is an interesting experiment designed to give you considerable insight into your brain and body's ability to learn new behaviors. Select an often-used door in your living space. Place a reminder sign on it saying, *left hand only*, i.e. if the left is your lesser used hand. Every time you open or close the door, use the lesser-used hand. It will be awkward at first then slowly you will get used to it. That getting used to it, means that the brain is being reorganized to accommodate your desire to open and close the door with you left hand. Your brain is becoming more ambidextrous. The outcome is that both hands now "know" how to do the job. They know because your brain has new patterns that control your hands. We are amazingly pliant. All we have to do is assiduously practice the behaviors we want. Begin with small things, and take pride in your ability to control your learning process. Become the little train that could . . . and did. Your self-worth will benefit in the process.

My personal interest in Ambidexterity is with juggling. Juggling has attracted scientific curiosity. An example is: the Beek and Lewbel study, *The Science of Juggling: Studying the Ability to Toss and Catch Balls and Rings Provides Insight into Human Coordination, Robotics and Mathematics.* A more popular look at juggling is the 1994 Gelb and Buzan book, *Lessons from the Art of Juggling.*

The Great Good of Failure

There's an old saying, "Success is a failure turned inside out." The inside of failure is a good place to find the road to success. The inside of failure invites exploration. Please know there is always some good in failure. When denial of failure is extensive, this prevents us from learning from it. The task is to look failure in the eye and treat it as a mere momentary event. Events and behaviors that bring on failure can be reduced. We all have the ability to learn from our failures.

KAT object manipulation activities make mistakes inevitable. But here is the good news, the more often you honestly make mistakes, the more quickly you learn what to do and what not to do. Hint: don't practice the mistake. Rather, constantly practice with the image of your goal in mind. *Discouragement is never an option.* Both trial and error are active ingredients in learning anything. You will see how this philosophy comes into play in KAT practice for better balance.

Rhythm, Cadence and Timing

All matter and processes in the universe possess their own characteristic rhythm, cadence or timing. Our heartbeat is a pulse, our footfalls must be properly timed to prevent falls, and we are safer when we stay in tune with environment rhythms. The regularity of our spinning earth is the basis of our measurement of time. We honor time when we practice staying within biological health boundaries. For example, fitness training is best scheduled three days a week. We need those in-between days for recovery. Rhythm, Cadence and Timing can be considered biological powers.

Music and Metronomes

Obviously, both music and a metronome have a beat. Both help the body and mind to focus on the outside world. Concentration on a rhythmic beat teaches us to control our responses within the confines of the beat. Dancing illustrates the body's ability to respond with rhythmic movement. Movement with music or a metronome is high-level *attentional-muscular-fuctional* interaction between our audio and motor systems.

Music and a metronome are great spurs to attention. But there are big differences in the way music and the metronome stimulate the central nervous system. A musical beat is more or less masked by the melody, counter point, etc. Also, music activates emotion. A metronome supplies only an austere, unadorned beat along with a between-beat auditory silence. This periodic quietude encourages attention to direct itself inward. New motor skill learning requires significant undiluted inward concentration.

The metronome pulse is a vibration dot of sound interspersed by deafening silences. Each dot of sound becomes a point of concentration. The beat is similar to a magnifying glass systematically concentrating sunlight to a point of white-hot light.

Focused by a metronome beat, or mesmerizing thought the human mind becomes white-hot in its ability to "see", i.e., (attend). KAT tools focus the attention ability of the central nervous system to improve itself. All we have to do is continually learn and practice new things and expect to become better.

Poetry has meter, meter means rhythm, rhythm means a beat, and the beat is an external stimulus, which spurs a central nervous system response. Staying within the beat is rather like following the rules of the road. Follow the rules of balance and you will be safe.

During metronome silences, we are given time to explore feelings, internal muscle tensions, and/or pockets of anxiety, all while practicing a Kinetic Arts skill. Whatever you do, such as walking, counting, winking, fingers snapping, reciting poetry, singing, or dancing, do it to a beat. As you read the next chapter on Tools, you will see many ways you can use a beat to make your practice more interesting, fun, and balance enhancing. Allow rhythmic generated time to guide your behavior. The benefit? Keeping in time to the beat will make you more aware of the rhythms that your body needs to retain its health and balance.

I am adamant about the benefits of movement synchronized to an exterior rhythmic beat. Why? From the beginning of society, human beings have danced and sung. Rhythmic cadence is part of our very being. The human bio-package responds to the power of rhythm. Rhythm moves us physically, emotionally and mentally. After all, the entire Universe is rhythmic. Our clock and bio-time is based on the movement of our earth. Seconds are but units of earth spin. It is not surprising we earth beings need and love rhythm in all it forms.

Kai Bhi

The term Kai Bhi is a take-off of Tai Chi. The K is for Kinetic and the B is for Balance. Tai Chi has been around for a long time. It is a wonderfully formalized, healthful routine, especially good for balance. Kai Bhi is different from Tai Chi in that it offers an added neurological benefit. Kai Bhi uses hand-held objects, which accentuates the need to keep in touch with the outside world. Object(s) are transferred from hand to hand with each movement cycle. The objects are rarely tossed from one hand to the other; there is only a gentle, and very conscious transfer between the two hands. This is in keeping with the peaceful, controlled movement patterns inherent in Tai Chi.

A simple example of Kai Bhi is the KAT V exercise, outlined in the next chapter under Ball Warm Ups. A ball is passed from hand to hand in a variety of patterns, all while rocking from side to side. The Lazy 8 exercise is another example. (See the next section under Lazy 8.)

Toss-Catch-Interval (TCI)

Mystery is in the air! There is something magically appealing about tossing an object into the air and catching it again. The skill needs considerable practice to master it. But I am biased, because as a juggler of 65+ years, I've initiated millions of tosses and catches. Until a few years ago, I never thought much about it. It was just juggling. But after studying neurology, I find that a great deal of incredible neurology is occurring during this brief interval when the object is in the air. I call this airtime, the *Toss-Catch-Interval.* It is a distinctive element of KAT.

During the toss-catch-interval, the object is not under human control. Rather, it is controlled by the force of gravity, the density of the air, the weight and shape of the object and the force with which the object was tossed. To successfully catch an object, our nervous system must adjust to these conditions. Not until it is caught again does it come back under human command. If previous tossing and catching experience is lacking, learning will be difficult. However, when the nervous system is challenged with new learning, it meets the challenge by learning the skill. The journey to any success is via practice.

KAT equipment provides the challenge. Your task is to progress toward tool manipulation mastery, which is the primary responsibility of the upper body. As the upper body proceeds toward control of a tool, the rest of the body is responsible for the control of balance. When one body part becomes better, all parts benefit. The process also enhances and extends attention, confidence, and general fitness. Repeated trial and error enhances the capacity to persist.

During the interval between the toss and the catch, attention is 'magically' magnified. This of course is not magic; rather it is the felt need to intensely focus on catching the object. After all, we tossed it, we are duty bound to catch it.

Immeasurable neurological wizardry transpires during the Toss-Catch- Interval. When the skill is repeatedly practiced, new neural patterns are created. These new pathways, even in an incomplete form, stimulate the body toward a more graceful performance, which in turn sets the stage for the brain to become more organized. As the brain becomes more integrated, motor control is heightened. Trial and error is the medium in which this happens. Brain-body reciprocity is a beautiful example of cooperation for the purpose of willful control.

Children are a state of hyper-attentiveness most of the time. They need a lot of sleep in order to recover from the vast amounts of energy they use in thinking, doing, and learning. For children the entire world is strange and new. They want to do what others can do and they are driven by their instincts to learn. Hyper-attentiveness is the optimum learning state. The trick for adults is to never give into age, i.e., retain that zest of childhood forever.

Direct and Peripheral Vision

When we look at an object in a concentrated manner, we are using our direct vision. Some call this "hard focus." But there is a soft focus too, which is peripheral vision. This is our side vision where we can see movement but have less definition for details. Normally we use both direct and peripheral vision. We need both for skill practice. The relationship between the two is necessary for good balance.

In the next chapter, you will notice that peripheral vision is mentioned along with many of the tools. This speaks to the importance of peripheral vision for stable balance.

Home Play

We Kinetic Artists never work: we play. KAT play is an array of focused commitments to health. Playful learning is fun when you know that the benefits of play are life enhancing and even life saving. Keep several of the KAT tools handy so you can use them for many short practice sessions. Do not allow boredom to creep in. (The next chapter will give you many tools to explore.)

In a sense, life is but a stage play.
I audaciously paraphrase Shakespeare by stating:
Life is our play and we play as the only player in it.

Mistakes and Trial and Error

Mistakes are good. The more often you make safe honest mistakes, the faster you learn. Mistakes keep you humble. Love your mistakes, and you will love yourself more when your goals are achieved. Discouragement is never an option. Practice is the process from inability to mastery.

A mistake is the error part of trial and error. When you give up there is no trial. No trial, no mistake, no learning. The trick is to try safely so any error is never catastrophic. Mistakes in the pursuit of learning show you have some healthy passion left.

When you learn anything new you become smarter. The brain, after all is a trial and error mechanism. Learning changes the brain's neurological patterns. New brain templates guide your body to perform more successfully. Trial and error is a biologically valid learning mode for both mental and physical learning.

Please don't think that you're half-baked.
The error after trial is never a mistake.
Take error in stride, go along for the ride.
What you derive is your carrot cake.

or
I often feel bad 'bout errors and mistakes.
I'm eternally squeezed by my attitudinal snakes.
But I kept on tryin'
and soon I'm a-flying,
above and beyond my self-limiting gait.

Note: Practice is trial 'n error's grandparents. Trial 'n error's parents are the power of will. Trail 'n error boosts of two coaches, one is persistence, and the other is patience. The act of trial 'n error energizes you as a get-up-and-do person.

Every time you try a new experiment you learning more.
You can't learn less.
Fuller

Patience, persistence and will-powered practice
open the floodgates of joy
with the force of learning.

Laughter

The Universe is a very serious place, after all there is just one of it. But our world is also a very silly place. How is this known? Because we are built to laugh. I conclude that I can laugh at anything . . . that doesn't hurt others. The moral is that KAT tricks may look silly on the surface, But, and this is a big BUT, if something like a yo-yo or tying a knot will build my brain so that I can balance better, then lead me to it. I plan to laugh a lot on the day I die, knowing I've done all I could do to remain independently mobile and balanced. By the way, laughter has been found to reduce pain, enhance immune levels, sharpen perspective, and most of all, laughter makes us the life of our own party . . . with the emphasis on LIFE.

Let me add a bit of a conversation with a philosopher friend. He said, "during the first half of our lives we think we're immortal, do what others tell us, and wrestle with our demons. If and when we conquer these, the second half of our lives, all we do is . . .
l-a-u-g-h.

Relaxation

Occasionally both body and mind need calming. A relaxed but attentive mind is good for learning. During longer practice sessions, take frequent mini-breaks. These are defined as mentally and physically turning in a different direction, i.e. relieving tension in the hands by shaking, taking a deep breath and blowing it out, jogging in place, and/or purposefully thinking about something else for a few seconds. Relaxation can be thought of as doing something different. Variety does have spice. Learning is better accomplished in short learning sessions.

One 90-year-old class member said that the class made her tired and afterwards she had to take a nap. But in just two weeks, she was stronger and gave up her nap. Her practice had become less tiring because she had learned to relax even while practicing. Building a better brain is tiring at first, but the challenge is worth it.

You will never enter the state of ease
unless you can count the petals in a breeze.

Herbert Benson in his 1975 book *Relaxation Response* helped to bring the concept of relaxation and the sphere of meditation together. As a Psychologist, he scientifically proved the many healthful physiological benefits of meditation. His book is simple to follow and still on the market.

Perspective

We are often so bound up (rigidified); in our past conditioning, we can't see any possibility of betterment. Under these hypnotized-like conditions, we have a difficult time seeing anything from a new perspective.

A new perspective, for many people, is that the body and mind are capable of becoming better. And there is no hope for change unless a new perspective is found. You and your brain are powerful actors on a stage where you can edit the script, change the scenery, be the star, and at the same time sit in the audience and enjoy your own one-person show.

This exercise will help you visualize what a new perspective looks like. In your own home you are going to experience something few people see. The object here is to make sure that you know there are different ways of looking and doing than you ever thought possible.

Lie on your back with your head in the corner of a room. Look up at three lines, one vertical and the other two at odd angles at the ceiling-wall juncture. This view has been there since the room was built. You knew it was there but never bothered to look at in this way. After this experience you will never seen any corner in the same way again. New experiences generate new perspectives. An up to date balance perspective will allow you to negate the danger of potholes. The world is full of new things to see and feel and learn from. Open up, the world is an exciting teacher . . . let the sunshine in.

Interactive Metronome Therapy

Interactive Metronome Therapy (IMT) is a computerized rehabilitation approach to testing and improving neurological connections within the brain. IMT therapy connects audio brain centers with the motor centers, with the additional value of augmenting attention capacity. IMT is assistive in working toward a more balanced brain. Master musicians and athletes use IMT to perfect their timing, as brain-injured patients who want to normalize their wayward brain circuits. In the next chapter your will see that there are many non-computerized ways reach the same goals.

Neuro-feedback Therapy

Neuro-feedback therapy is a computerized approach designed to help a person regain the proper ratio between the beta and theta (EEG) brain rhythms. When this is achieved, the brain returns to normal brain functioning. Practitioners are usually psychologists and less often psychiatrists. They report that the method to works well with a variety of conditions. Much more detail at: www.eegspectrum.com/FAQ/ or google neurofeedback for more.

Creative Regression (CR)

Mood control is a large part of your ability to learn. Let's put this in context. Children learn more per minute than adults. But wonderfully, some adults retain their youthful learning ability into old age. It's important to know that it can be done. A second factor is staying in touch with those good feelings of childhood. Here's a suggestion to all KAT students.

When you step through any classroom door, or any learning situation, 'become' the best child learner you ever were. An easy way to pinpoint your best memories is to review your elementary school years from 1th to 6th grade. Then judge which year was your best for learning, excitement, interest, health, teacher, etc. You may decide on the year when you had that genius teacher who made you feel special. Whatever your criteria, bring that feeling to any learning experience, especially to balance class. Learning is better accomplished when you feel expectant, joyful, youthful, and exuberant. Fun comes less from a particular activity than the mood with which you approach the activity. Come to class, or any life experience expecting to have fun. You can recover much of that childlike zest and zeal, and channel it in a mature manner. Creative Regression is a way of going back in order to move forward. And oh yes, forward is a life worth living.

Controlled Limitations or Constraint Therapy

The concept of Controlled Limitations is an outgrowth of a child development technique called Limitation of Space and Tools. When there are too many toys, (stuff), children flit from one thing to another and never deeply explore the possibilities of one item. The remedy is to limit toys and space, which helps them focus their attention. This technique has relevance to the balance class. One item such as a ball or baton is used, directly and indirectly, for the entire class. I am always surprised by the many new ways students create to handle the item under these conditions.

Imagine this. You are given a small ball and told you must keep it hidden all day long. This idea comes from magician Penn, of Penn and Teller. In an interview, Penn said that when he was in high school he would palm a small ball all day long without anyone knowing he had it. His goal was to diligently practice his slight-of-hand skill even while engaged in all his school activities. No wonder some people are good at what they do; they practice all day long.

Penn's constant practice helped me update on the concept of controlled limitations. Since 1990, medical professionals and psychologists have developed a technique called Constraint Therapy. This therapeutic technique is used under scrupulous medical supervision. Patients with neurological impairments, (such as brain injury or a stoke) such as paralysis on the right arm are constrained with a sling on their other arm. For many hours of therapy per day, they are given graded tasks to perform, using only their impaired side. Research suggests they progress quickly under this regime of intense concentration, constant practice, high motivation, and expert therapy. Constraint Therapy is also called Massed Practice.

This same concept is used in KAT. For instance, to improve coordination in the lesser-used arm and hand, place your good arm in a sling. Or you can put your good hand around your back and tuck your hand under your belt. Here, in no uncertain terms, you are using Controlled Limitation to force the impaired hand to practice. Necessity *is* the mother of invention. To accomplish the massed practice element, work the lesser side repeatedly during the day, the more often, the better.

A good example of Controlled Limitations is the previously stated opening a door with only your lesser-used hand. Others may be washing dishes, doing simple house chores, shaking hands, or even attempting to write, and all with an idle good hand. Frustration will be your first emotion, but even a little success will give the realization that practice is a reliable teacher.

Affirmations

Too often, the human mind drives itself into a self-defeating, downward spiral of self-doubt. Depression often follows. Positive affirmations encourage an upward spiral. Affirmations are honest, consciously crafted, positive statements designed to be repeated again and again. Positive thoughts crowd out negative thoughts. William James, a turn-of-the-century psychologist, advised, (I paraphrase), If you feel down, recall a past positive activity, example, like bowling. Then purposefully go bowling with a friend and be reminded of the good times. Positive behaviors and their underlying thoughts influence the mind, just as negative behavior hurls a person toward oblivion.

An especially powerful time to repeat affirmations is in the evening just before you drop off to sleep and in the morning just after you have awakened. But any other time is good for giving yourself a positive boost. Try the follow affirmation at least 20 or more times a day. *Every day, in every way, I am getting better and better.*

Say it aloud and find its rhythm. Then add some meaningful and fun gestures. You become the choreographer and the performer, as well as the main beneficiary of your own word power. Repetition need not be boring. When you really listen, you will plumb deeper levels of meaning. Affirmations can pull you up by your own bootstraps. We are a paradox; we own our troubles as well as our cures. We are the patient and the therapist. Affirmational words and their meaning, challenge the central nervous system to change toward the better you desire. And facing challenges is what Kinetic Arts health is all about.

The appendix has a few more good affirmations, including Rapp's Rap, which is a most positive affirmation with choreography. Memorize it and put Rapp's Rap to the test.

Hart's Five Characteristics of the Human Brain

They are: *Aggressive, Gaited-Gated, Talk, No Threat, and Trial and Error.* Memorize them as a constant reminder of the characteristics of healthy brain. The brain chapter has previously laid out these five in greater detail.

The Gottlieb Learning Scale

Ray Gottlieb is one of the few behavioral optometrists in the country. He has developed a unique five-point scale of the learning process. He uses his scale to help the mentally handicapped, brain injured, athletes, and even budding concert pianists to progress to their next higher level of ability. He encourages learners to place themselves on this five-point scale, and then take the challenge to move on to the next higher level.

Gottlieb's scale is in the form of five questions. The learning content is irrelevant.

1. Can I do it?
2. Can I do it well?
3. Can I do it well for a long time?
4. Can I do it well for a long time in the face of distraction?
5. Can I do it creatively?

When you know where you are on this scale, you will better understand what and how to practice to reach the next level. The first three levels are reached with the help of two friends, trail and error, and their soul mate, persistence. But the fourth level needs some explanation. The fourth level requires an added approach.

Here are a couple of ideas. Practice your activity while focusing across the room. Notice that you are doing the activity with only the use of your peripheral vision. Make it harder by doing it in front of a mirror and concentrating on the mirror image. Try multi-tasking, such as spelling words out loud as your practice your activity. Or say a poem, or sing a song, or perform any task that uses a different part of the brain. The distraction might be someone waving his or her arms in front of you as you perform. The point of stage four is simple, to better learn to pay full attention to what your want to do. Learning comes faster that way.

The fifth level, creativity, is defined here as doing your thing, in your own way, with style, verve, and enthusiastic pizzazz. A unique personality is worth developing. If you don't think you have any personality for the activity, then, *fake* it, pizzazz is healthy. Remember Art Carney and Jackie Gleason. (See the paragraph on Creativity below.)

Intelligence

Intelligence, beginning with conscious and all form of awareness, is a large part of balance. Be smart, don't try to do things on the edge of your ability when you feel down, out of sorts, or angry. All these states of mind heighten emotions that obscure learning. Under these negative conditions, the brain is prevented from doing what it usually can do easily. Hint: perform a repetitive, unthinking activity and the stress will subside. Examples might be: sweeping, raking, walking or mowing the yard.

Intelligence is characterized by awareness of your negatives, then doing something about them so your positives may shine. Be aware of your negatives and face the reality of the damage they can do. The human condition is far from perfect but we can do much to correct, control, and cure ourselves. The real you is your will power and it can be strengthened. Dogged persistence is one side of control; the other is to register stressful events, then respond with logic rather than emotion. Intelligence, to a large degree, is control of the self and all that entails.

Groups

The group is a powerful force within itself. *Esprit de corps* is the name we give to group solidarity. That feeling of cohesion comes from interpersonal support, responsibility, motivation and oneness of purpose. This is one reason working in a class group is rewarding. People help each other just by being there. The old adage that people need people is true. (The next chapter treats groups as a tool.)

Foot Wear

Remember when we joked about the *little old lady in tennis shoes*? The modern tennis shoes have come a long way. Now they look better, fit better, and are more accepted in public. They also greatly disallow slippage. Fall prevention is the goal. A firm understanding is good under any circumstance.

Creativity

There's a funny thing about the human brain: it, i.e. (we) can do more than we ever thought possible. Again and again, KAT suggests that each person can dream up all kinds of exercises that stimulate the brain and body to do better and better. Solving any problem that comes across your life is a good starter. The KAT axiom says this in no uncertain terms. *Do what you can, then a little bit more.* Keep your options open, search for possibilities, investigate, explore, seek out, and discover yourself anew each and every new day. You were born out of a very creative process. You have lost it, *only* if you think you have lost it.

Cross Training

The concept of Cross Training was introduced to me in the form of an aphorism by a Physical Education instructor in the 1940s. He said, "You learn to play baseball in the winter while playing basketball and learn to play basketball in the summer while playing baseball." In explanation, both basketball and football require similar basic skills, such as running, catching, following rules, staying alert, and all the while staying well balanced.

All action sport participation requires movement and continual skill enhancement. Thus, we learn to do a lot of specific movements such as throwing and catching from many different activities. No learned motor, knowledge or motivational skill is ever wasted. Said dramatically with balance in mind:

Every cell in the body either contributes to
or detracts from your ability to balance.

You never know which skill will save you from a fall. The more you know and can do, the more you can learn and learn to do.

KAT uses the concept of Cross Training by promoting brain pathway integration. It is the melding together of different motor skills that renders the brain more whole and balanced. The levels of brain integration build on each other. There does not seem to be any end to where this process can take you.

The mastery of each KAT tool and activity demands a unique neural response. The more varied the skills that your body and brain acquire, the more immune you are to falls. KAT tools provide a variety of practice opportunities.

Neuroplasticity

In the last quarter of the 21st century, the brain has become a ringing research refrain. However, betterment of the brain has been an evolutionary matter, an educational matter, a personal matter of reason, logic and emotion, and not to leave out, a political matter (as with propaganda and brain washing),

Man has always known that there was something within him or her that possessed the ability to learn. I don't mean to make the brain less that it is, but one thing is simple: *When anything is learned, something in you has changed,* i.e. the brain is altered. Behavior, (performance), is the outward manifestation of this brain ability. But the ability to learn and adjust is greater than commonly understood. Just in the last ten years researchers have discovered many of the intricacies of memory, intra brain commutations, and how best to grow a good brain. Neuroscience calls this life-long brain ability to rework itself, *neuroplasticity.* It is defined by Jeffery Schwartz as, "the ability of neurons to forge new connections, to blaze new paths through the cortex, even to assume new roles. In shorthand, neuroplasticity means rewiring of the brain ".

Schwartz in his book, The *Mind and the Brain,* goes beyond the brain to postulate a distinct difference between the mind and the brain. The mind is where the real you, the inner you, resides and has it being. As a Psychiatrist, he simplifies his picture of mind by saying that it contains four powerful forces. These forces work together and can change the brain's wiring that carries out what the mind determines.

These four have been mentioned previously. However, I dare not apologize for the repetition because the mere knowing of these four is a kind of personal research facility which can lead to better use of your magnificent human capabilities that are you. First is *attention* which gives thought focus. Needed is direction which is supplied by *intention.* But these two go nowhere without the power inherent in the concept of *volition.* Now the three, attentional focus, intentional direction, plus volitional power, all together create the fourth attribute of the mind, the power of *will.* Without these four working together, the mind is a slave of the brain, when it should be the other way around.

When I point my mind, it is this that I find.
I get what I earn and earn what I learn,
that my body and mind, are always entwined.

Attention, intention, volition and will can be bolstered by perseverance of motor skill learning. The body and the mind-brain interact reciprocally to strengthen each other. Because biology needs periodic reminding, i.e. prompting, it is life-long work, but worth the effort to become the person you know you really can be. Schwartz is not original in these thoughts. He echoes William James writing from the 1890s. James book is Psychology*: A Briefer Course.* 1892. It is still in print.

The next chapter gives a broad array of physical tools which will help you achieve your goal of lifelong balance.

Kinetic Arts Training Tools and Suggested Usage

Tools are like pools.
Both are fluid in nature.
Either may be benign,
or be wave-like.
But one thing is sure,
both nurture body and soul,
only . . . when rightly used.

Introduction to KAT Tools

When primitive humans discovered tools, their use and manipulation made the human brain grow in size and complexity. Progress, in any sense of the word, relies on tools. This section offers details about how to use KAT tools to enhance your balance, your brain, and your well-being.

Tools are the pulse of Kinetic Arts Training. The neurological challenge provided by the manipulation of each tool is unique. Each tool contains distinct properties and functions. Your brain responds to motor learning challenges by creating new brain connections and pathways. These new brain pathways become control templates for facilitating better balance. Your purpose is to build a better brain, which facilitates better balance. Tool manipulation is the bridge. This is one case where the path and purpose are synonymous. There seems to be no end to what the brain can learn.

Quite literally, KAT practice is the process of discovering the needed action to properly manipulate a KAT tool. Even a small bit of mastery reorganizes your brain. You will realize this change as your skill mastery improves. Each improved new brain template, in turn, facilitates a corresponding improvement in the skill. With repeated practice, the skill gradually becomes more automatic. Now the higher learning centers may devote themselves to learning new challenges. With more connections and pathways in the brain, the better your needs are served. And balance is a constant need.

The term *tool* is broadly used to mean an object, philosophy, activity, body part, body function, motivation, friend, or your own willpower. KAT tools are designed to enhance the many components of balance, which are:

Agility
Balance
Centering
Concurrency
Coordination
Reaction time
Self-confidence

Mental concentration
Attention augmentation
Direct and peripheral visions
Eye-hand-brain coordination
Cross brain-lobe communication
Power, especially lower body strength
Imaginative and goal focusing

Warning: You may become addicted to the health aspects inherent in Kinetic Arts Training tools. However, some addictions are very positive. Any repeated activity can become a *healthy* addiction when is it is *legal, inexpensive, and healthy.*

Here we go with a few KAT tools. Some will turn you on more than others. Choose the ones you like, and then stay with them until they are mastered. While you are practicing, look for the principle involved in their manipulation. For instance, a heavy ball takes more muscle strength to toss than a lighter one. However, a ball that is very light, like a crumpled sheet of paper, will not activate the muscles in the arm and thus must be sensed only by the eyes and the surface nerves on the palm of the hand. Both heavy and light are useful.

Beanbags

A beanbag is nothing more than a squishy ball. They don't roll away when dropped, and they are great for tender hands. Even children can make one. They can be stuffed with beans or corn or anything that adds the desired size and weight. Round ones are best for easy handling.

A *penny ball* can be easily made. Stack about eight or nine pennies on a sheet of paper. Then crumple the paper into a ball around the pennies. Put a couple of strips of tape around and you have a nice weighted ball. Obvious joke: have a ball, cheap and convenient.

Beanbag Jacks

Jacks is a great old game. If you have not played Jacks for a long time, start by using beanbags in place of the usual rubber ball as well as the jacks. The beanbag won't bounce, so merely toss the bag into the air, scoop up the other beanbags with the same hand, and then catch the beanbag. When you get the hang of it with your best hand, try the other hand. Always begin new skill learning in the easiest way to assure some initial success.

Ball Warm-Ups: Propeller, Elevator, V, and Crab

These four ball warm-up exercises can be performed with one ball, a beanbag or almost any thing you can toss and catch. All four exercises provide many balance enhancers. Your ball (or object,) should be small enough to be easily held. A tennis ball is too large for most hands, but can be used. The ball is a marvelously useful tool for stimulating the nervous system. One fun definition of a ball is:

A ball is a tool, a toy, a treasure.
It's valuable and enjoyable beyond measure.
You can use it at play in your leisure.
Or you can work it for balance and reap great pleasure.

The Propeller Hold a ball or beanbag in the fingers of your best hand. Hold the ball at nose height with the other hand directly below it. Release the ball so it drops straight down to the waiting hand. To assure success, the flight of the ball can be short at first. But as your skill grows, your hands can be moved farther apart. First, use your right hand to drop the ball, and then try the left. Alternate the dropping–catching hands. Try to perform this propeller action in a fixed rhythm (which is one of the goals of all KAT skills). Later you can toss and catch a ball, from hand to hand, in a simple trajectory

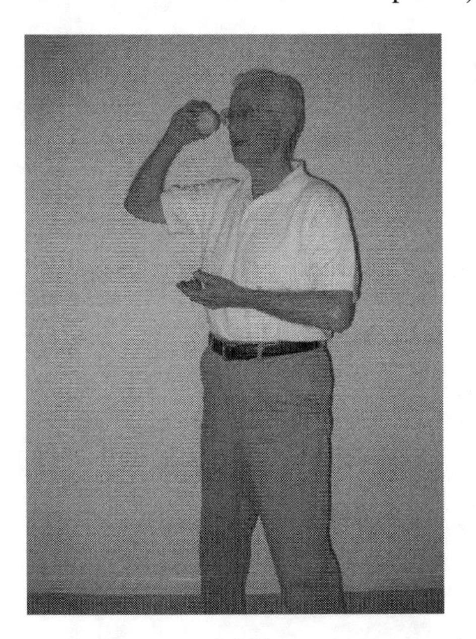

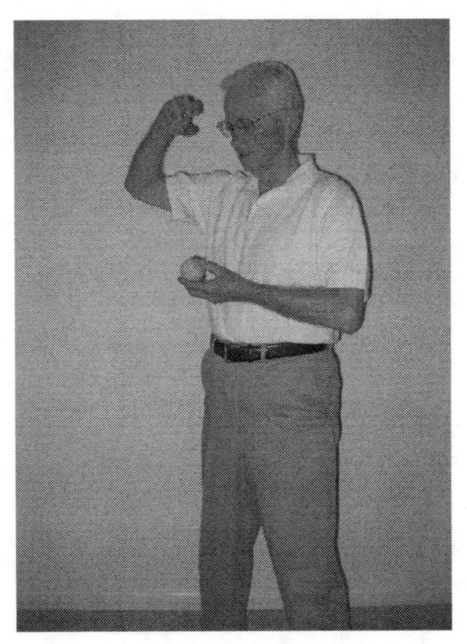

Confidence grows as your skill grows. Remember, mistakes are good. Learn from them. The brain is a trial-and-error mechanism. Soon, as you grow in skill and confidence, the distance between the two hands may be increased. The dropping distance is a measure of proficiency.

Novice catchers too often try to catch a ball in the palm or even on the heel of their hand. This strategy makes it necessary to trap the ball with the fingers. The difficulty is that even a beanbag often bounces off the palm before the fingers can trap it. A helpful strategy is to curl the fingers into a kind of web-like first baseman's mitt and catch the ball in your finger web. With finger-web catching, the ball does not have to be trapped and it is immediately ready to be directed into the next toss.

Make a conscious effort to consider just what you are doing with your eyes. Experiment to find the best use of your vision. It might be difficult to keep your eye on the ball if the ball is too close for proper eye focus. Solve the problem by moving the ball away from your face for better focus. Much later, you can try the propeller with eyes closed. Marvelously, most people are surprised at how well they can work blind after only a few trials.

I ask students to put a little personal style into their actions. KAT style is any mode of movement that renders the activity more personal and fun. A healthful emotional release leaps forth with the injection of personality into your performance. Now you can honestly say, 'I've got it all together'. . . at least for now.

Add a little complexity. As the right hand is being extended up, and before the ball has been dropped, rock your body to the left, placing extra weight on the left foot. Drop the ball and reverse the action to the right. This makes the propeller like a full-body coordinated dance move. Put as much weight on one leg as is safe for you. The more your knees are bent the more you are exercising your quadriceps, which are the front thigh muscles. The stronger your quads are, the more upright, balanced posture is assured. You might want to say, practice makes the propeller go round.

Later, you can focus on a distant object while doing the propeller. This exercises your peripheral vision, which is also an important part of balance. The eyes are 30 to 40 percent of your balance. But, when the eyes are closed, the vestibular and the somatosensory systems do the best they can to take over the visual function. Students are continually surprised by what their body and mind can do.

An even higher level of skill is demonstrated when the propeller is performed in the face of distraction, such as standing in front of a mirror while performing. It takes energy and practice to disregard unimportant sensory information. One way to learn to ignore distraction is to rhythmically perform the propeller as you turn, bit by bit, around in a circle. You can make the exercise even more exacting by designating a specific number of propeller drops to accomplish in one full revolution. As skill in any motor action increases, so does the ability to attend. Why? Because you are increasing your concentration by learning what *not* to do as well as what to do. Practice makes the skill better, along with the ability to attend.

Another variation for the propeller is to set the goal of a certain number of repetitions. When you have achieved your goal, increase your expectation. It is important to push your body and mind, which will make you more durable, stronger and able to handle the intricacies of upright locomotion. You never know when an emergency will demand that you react with exacting agility and certitude. Please be ready.

The ultimate propeller can be done with the upper hand stretched high above the head, while the lower catching hand is stretched all the way below the waist. But start with your hands close together. The ability to concentrate and attend also declines with age, disuses and disease. This is biological reality. However, when people face reality, they become motivated to keep themselves balanced and upbeat. You will notice that all KAT tools demand focused attention. Attention can be augmented along with learning a motor skill. Yes, your body and brain do have the ability to remain functional much longer than most of us think. But we must provide the desire and the will to conquer the apathy that too often prevails.

I have given many suggestions with regard to the propeller. All these basic ideas, such as the exercise of peripheral vision, personal style, eyes closed, and so on, are applicable to all KAT tools.

The Elevator Raise your empty hand high over your head with your palm up. The ball, in your lower hand, becomes an elevator and rises slowly to the waiting palm. Switch hands and repeat. This slow exchange is a freight elevator. You can play express elevator by tossing the ball from the basement up to the penthouse.

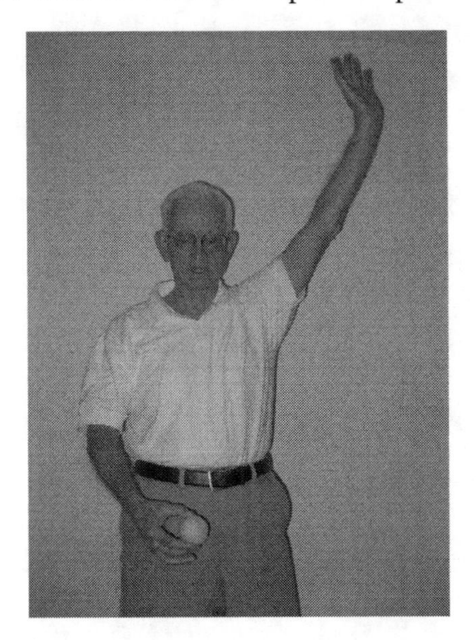

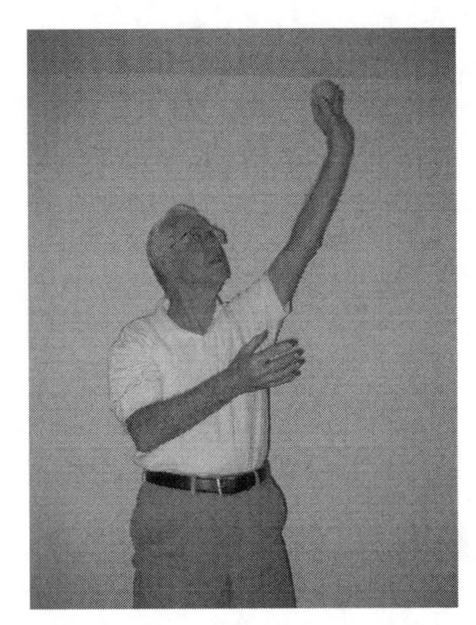

The elevator demands the full body to stretch itself upward. The action keeps the shoulder joints flexible. Believe it or not, shoulder flexibility is an important part of your balance.

As your elevator skill becomes better, you can sway back and forth with the rhythm of the action. Be sure your knees are bent. You should be able to feel the quads contract as you do this. This rocking motion is actually weight lifting. The weight of your body has just become a balance-strengthening tool. The elevator demands that both hands stretch to their maximum height at the moment the ball is exchanged. As you stretch upward, do so stretching upward through your legs, hips, abdomen, chest, and neck. You will find this to be a marvelous tool for good posture.

When you keep your eye on the ball as it goes up to the top hand, it is obvious you must tilt your eyes and neck upward. If you have vertigo, be careful of positioning your head upward. If vertigo is a concern, then first try the elevator with your back into a corner to assure safety.

The V Both hands are placed together in front of your body with a ball in the crux of your hands that form a V. Action begins from there. There are three basic V exercises.

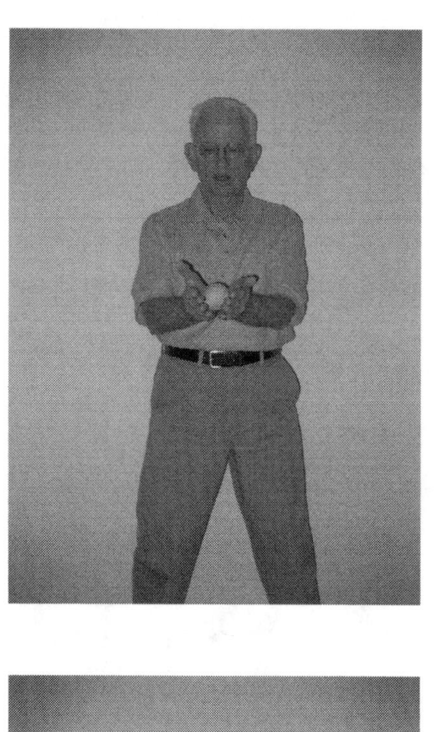

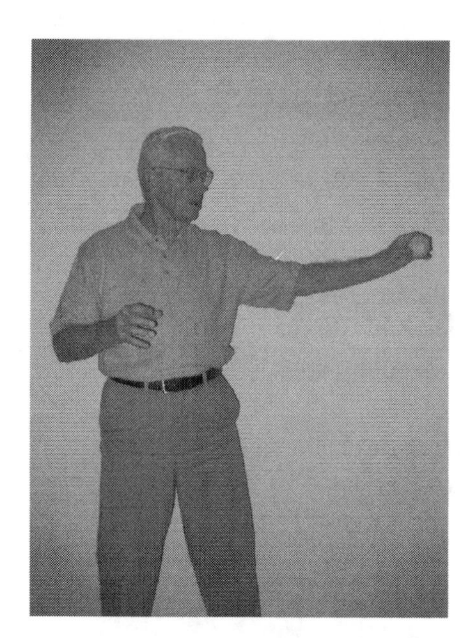

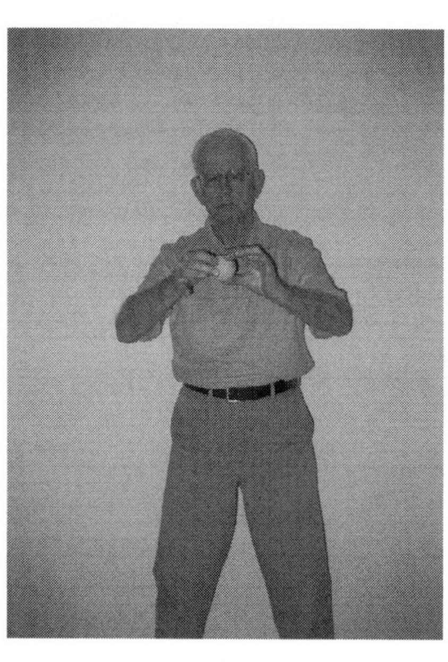

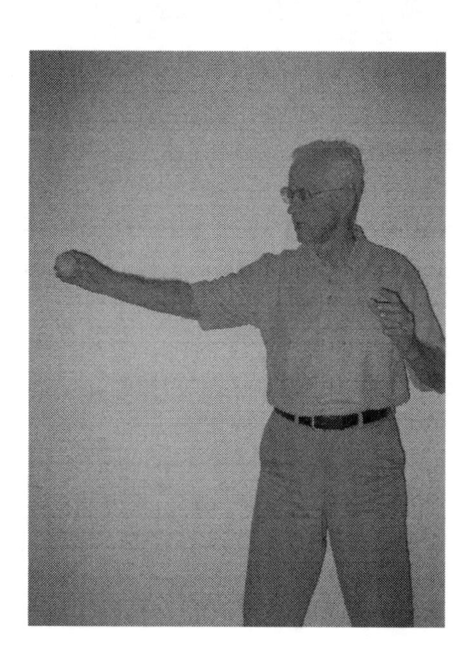

1, Side to side. Begin with your feet apart. Your left hand and arm move the ball horizontally to your left side as far out as you can reach. The ball is then slowly brought back to the center midline where the ball is transferred to the right hand that repeats the same action to the right side. As you extend all the way out to one side, lean far enough to that side so that most of your weight is on one foot. If you can place all your weight on that leg, then slightly lift the other. But, always be safe.

You will see the similarity between this V exercise and the slow, deliberative moves in Tai Chi. The difference is that, in KAT, there is a hand-held object that is passed from hand to hand to provide a dynamic point of concentration. To heighten mental awareness, move the ball in an M pattern or a W. Try writing your name in large cursive letters in the air. You are writing for yourself, not an audience. This means you will have to move from your left to right as you air-write in big letters. Notice that your feet must coordinate with your hand action. Good balance requires coordination from all parts of the body.

Think up your own patterns but remember that the V is always done slowly and with concentration. The goal is gracefulness and effortlessness. As you pass the ball from hand to hand, receive the ball with one fewer finger on each pass. Experiment with whatever it takes to extend your practice time and the accompanying concentration. Achievement of any goal requires both mental focus and physical practice.

2. Front to back. Place the ball in your right hand, then stretch it out to the front and slightly to the left. The left hand and arm are stretched out to the back. The two hands move slowly toward each other and meet at the left hip. When they meet, the ball is transferred to the left hand and the ball now moves back as the right arm moves forward. Your eyes should follow the ball, which means your must twist your neck, shoulders, spine and hips, while your feet remain solid. Keeping your knees bent helps the body twist more comfortably. The ball then comes back to the front and the pattern is repeated. Twisting is a range-of-motion exercise. Some forms of arthritis are kept at a minimum when you maximize the range of motion in your joints. Remember also to perform the front to back on the other side.

3. Alligator. Place the ball in your right hand keeping you elbow stiff and held down at a 45-degree angle in front. Your left arm and hand are held up diagonally in front at same angle. This is the alligator's open mouth. Bring your arms together (the alligator's mouth is now closed). The ball is transfer to your left hand, then the ball moves down as the empty right moves up. Keep your eyes on the ball as it goes up and down. As described, the right hand is always on the top. At some point, change your arm position so that your left hand is on top.

The Crab Usually our tossing and catching is from a supinated (palm up) position. The Crab is performed with the hand in a pronated (palm down) position. The elbow is bent at a right angle. As the hand moves up the ball is released. This upward action allows the ball to hang in the air a bit longer than if you just dropped it. Then come straight down and trap it in your hand. The crab is a continuous up-down hand-arm motion, going up to make the ball airborne, and coming down to catch it. Perform this at your own speed. The crab action is like catching flies, gnats or mosquitoes in your hands on a summer's day. Try the crab with both hands.

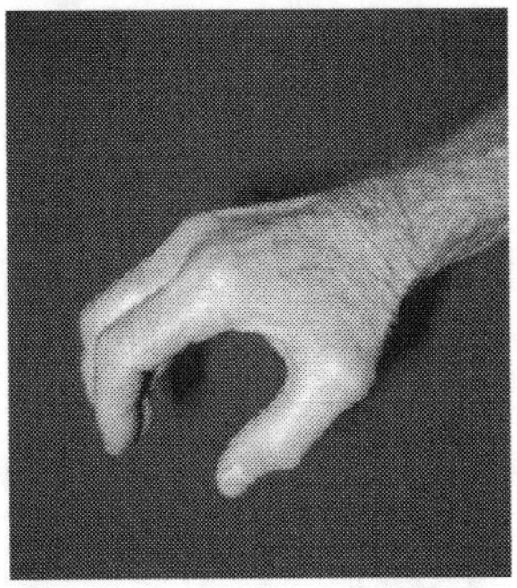

Some students have great difficulty with the crab action. I suggest that they hold the ball lightly as the hand goes up and when the hand comes down, tighten their fingers on the ball. This is an excellent preparation for the real air-borne crab. Soon you will feel the rhythm and are confident enough to let the ball become airborne.

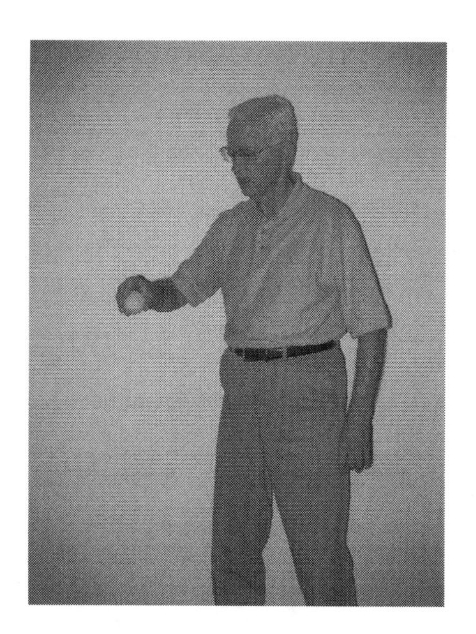

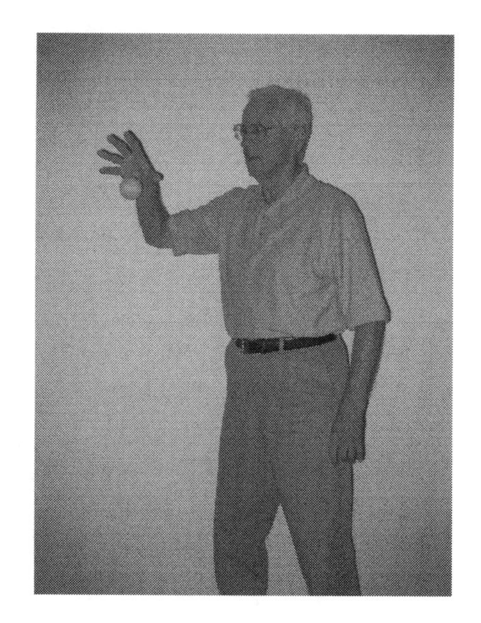

Crab Variations

- Walk while doing the crab. Catch the ball in time with each footfall. Vary the speed according to your skill.
- Turn around while crabbing. Count the number of steps you take the first time around, and then try to duplicate that exact number with the next turn around. When you achieve that number consistently, change the number and learn the new timing.
- Perform the crab while looking at a distant object. This is peripheral vision practice. (Peripheral vision practice can be done with all KAT tools.)
- Crab while walking through a self-made obstacle course. The course does not have to be elaborate. The rule of thumb is to challenge yourself with complexity, but not so much as to be unsafe.
- Stand on one leg while doing the crab. If this is impossible at first, hold on to the wall with your other hand, or stand in a corner on one leg while doing the crab.
- Using two balls, crab with both hands synchronously, and then alternately.
- Count for five crabbings, and then hum for five crabbings, all while keeping rhythm to the crab beat. Go back and forth between counting and humming.
- Spell words while crabbing. First, spell familiar words from memory. As each letter is pronounced aloud, crab the ball. Then continue through the word. The spaces between words also deserve a crab pulse. Spell the word forward, then backwards. Learning new words is faster and more fun when mental and physical actions are coordinated. New words can be written large on a paper or a blackboard, in front of you.
- Crab the ball in the air higher than usual; clap your hands before it is caught again. A variation is to pat your hips, with both hands, while the ball is in the air.
- Sing, walk, and crab all the way across the room as you crab.
- Crab to a musical beat as you walk. Then add counting, winking, snapping fingers, reciting poetry, singing, dancing to the beat—you get the idea. Allow a musical beat to guide your behavior. The benefit comes from the need to stay with the beat. The side effects are that you become more aware of the rhythms your body needs to keep its balance. Great attention is required to march in step with other people. Hand in-hand and stride-for-stride has its added pleasures, and all while crabbing.
- Create your own variations. All real crabs appreciate your interest.

Propeller, elevator, the V and the crab.
Drop it and lift it and sway and grab.
These actions will make your brain grow strong.
Keep on the move and you can never go wrong.

Note: With all age groups, I tell the story of how this crab action was discovered. Basketball dribbling is an obvious comparison. But there is a more imaginative story. I was walking on a beach and met a crab. The crab said that she had found a ball and invented a game. She suggested it would be good for my balance because I have only two legs. I named the action the Crab in honor of my friend, the talking crab. She was so proud of being found practical for something other than food.

Now, the non-myth version. As a kid, I learned to juggle. One juggling pattern was tossing and catching with palms down, a movement I now call the Crab. Truth may be truth, but fiction is more fun.

Ball Bouncing

Dribbling a basketball is a familiar activity. A cheap dime-store ball is good to bounce. Try it first using both hands to catch. Two hands are better than one. Then imagine yourself a pro basketball player and try it one-handed. Left and right dribbles are a good test. Taking a wide stance and bending your knees actually helps to control your dribbling.

Your spatial and reaction abilities are alive and well when you bounce a ball off a wall. Make it harder. Stand facing a corner and bounce a ball off one wall to the other, like a pool shot and catch it with the other hand. The ricocheting action, back and forth between hands, really makes your eyes and brain work. A different visual challenge comes when you bounce a lightweight ball off a mirror. This activity helps you determine how to use your eyes to differentiate the real ball from the reflected one. Success is a good reflection on you.

Ball in Spoon

Remember the child's racing game where an egg is placed in a spoon and the participants are asked to run without dropping the egg? I do not advocate a race, or an egg. Walking with a marble or ball or beanbag in a spoon will do fine. Vary your walking course. Try a zigzag pattern, walk fast or slow, and make circles, all at your own pace, of course. The ball-in-spoon exercise is good for learning to do more than one thing at a time. A chair bound person can gain a lot of eye-hand coordination without leaving their chair. All they have to do is move the spoon in front of them from side to side. Keep your eye on the ball.

Paddle Ball Bouncing

This can be done using the flat of your hand or a ping-pong paddle. Bounce the ball off the paddle, catch it with your other hand, and repeat. Change hands. Ping-pong is the great paddle game. Tennis is even more exacting. But if these are not possible, do what you can then always a little bit more.

Scarf

A scarf can be used much like a ball, except its floating nature makes it easier to use. Start with one scarf, toss it up with one hand and catch it with the other. Keep the palm of your hand down as with the crab. Watch the scarf as it folds and unfolds in beautiful flight. Try to control its gyrations with the way you release it in the air. Can you play with two scarves at a time? Toss and catch them in unison.

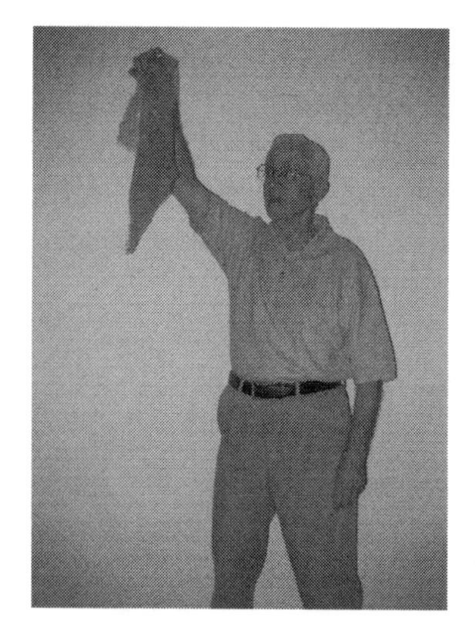
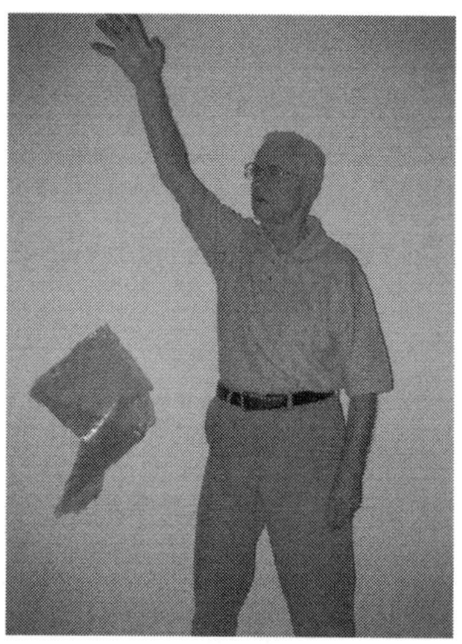
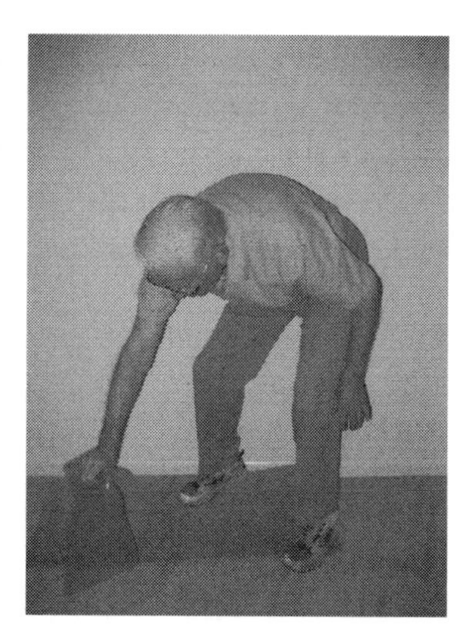

Then make the opposite pattern, right, then left, and repeat.

A hefty air conditioner can play havoc with a scarf. So, can a breeze outside. Find the best place to practice your scarf dance.

There are inexpensive scarves for juggling on the market. But a scarf can be made in your home for no money at all. Most grocery stores have gone from paper to plastic bags. One plastic bag will make three scarves. First, cut off the handles, and then slice down one side and then across the bottom. Now you have a long rectangular sheet of plastic. Cut this into three squares. You get three KAT toys for just a little effort. There are many things you can do with a scarf that just can't be done with other objects.

Try this. First, simply drop your scarf and let it float down. Catch it just before it touches the floor. This is good for balance and coordination, as well as exercising the inner ear. Keep going long enough and you will get a real workout. (It is ok to puff a little.) Be aware of how the scarf flows and gyrates in the air. If the scarf remains parallel to the floor, it will descend slowly but it does gyrate in its own peculiar way. Your adjustment ability is challenged. This simple drop can be coordinated with your stepping in place.

There are many ways to catch any object, including scarves. Think directionally. You can catch it with the palm up, palm down, as with the crab, then you can turn your palm to the right, then left as you catch it moving sideways. You might do this in a planned sequence, and to a musical beat. And don't forget the four diagonals, moving to the upper left and right, and lower left and right.

For a change of pace, fold the scarf in half, and then in quarters, and so on, until you have a tight little package. Test out to see how many folds it takes until it can't be folded any more. This is a good little game for children learning halves, fourths, eighths, sixteenths, and so forth.

It is also good for anyone who needs to exercise his or her fingers. Try crabbing the scarf "blind" and "see" its gyration with your mind's eye.

A scarf can be used for all four of the ball warm-up exercises. With any of these exercises, remember the KAT motto: *Do what you can, and then a little bit more.* Let's make the *little* in the motto practical. Walk in your usual manner with a scarf or object in your hand. Now walk with a little more vigor than usual, a little faster, a little harder, a little longer, with a bit larger steps, and all the while the ball or folded scarf is moving back and forth between hands. You could walk with a friend, while reciting a poem to the rhythm of your crabbing and walking. When you make the decision to add a little bit more to what you can already do, it becomes very personal. Personal is good. Your *little* reachable goals add up to better controlled movement. If no success comes right away, persist. Persistence is a character trait that will boost you to that better life where you deserve to be.

Counting

Counting can accompany any of the KAT exercises. For example, once you have learned to do the crab or the propeller, simultaneously count in rhythm with the action. Say the numbers loudly at the exact time the ball is caught. Not only voice volume but also, bigger-than-life pronunciation is encouraged. This is also true, for example, with the elevator. When you reach up high, (as for the stars), really reach. Limb and body extension, makes dancers so much fun to watch. You are the dancer. Your stage is your life. Live it tall.

Counting need not be boring. Vary the way you do it. When it becomes easy to count forward, count backwards. Count by twos, threes, and so forth. Count in a foreign language. Walk and count at the same time. Recite a poem, saying one word or syllable on each footfall. Words can be used like numbers.

Some people like to challenge their brain by doing calculations as they crab or just walk. With each footfall, say aloud the calculation, such as, 1+1 is 2. 2+2 is 4, 3 + 3 is 6, and on and on. Notice that each calculation is a five-count beat. When you get to the larger numbers the cadence changes. Here is another case of adjustment that you must work out. Multiplication or division makes it even more interesting.

Vary the task content. A lady told me she had 11 grandchildren. She listed their names in alphabetic order, Angela, Brian, and so forth, then memorized the list and repeated them forward and backward in time with her footfalls. For added challenge, she repeated the number, followed by the name as they appeared on the list, such as, one – Angela, etc. When she had conquered this level she would say the even number, then the odd and in other combinations. Now she reordered the 11 names by age. This woman was creatively personal with her practice. There must be a million ways to stimulate your brain and walk at the same time. This is a great concurrency exercise. (See the walking section below for more possibilities).

Singing adds another dimension. Try walking and singing one word or syllable for each footfall. Can't you hear Julie Andrews singing:

"Doe, a deer, a female deer. Ray, a drop of golden sun.
Me, a name I call myself. Fa a long long way to run.
So, a needle pulling thread. La, a note that follows So.
Ti, a drink with jam and bread. And that brings us back to doe."

Brains are designed to learn. Learning pays off in added skill, enhanced alertness, and greater ability to pay attention to your balance. You will never be bored when you insist on learning more and more.

Walking

Just plain walking is great for balance. But walking can be made even more productive by purposefully challenging the brain to build new brain pathways while moving from point A to B. Here are some suggestions.

First, remember that it is five or more feet from the top of the head to the bottom of the feet. Let's say you decide to move. Your eyes see where you wish to go, your brain sends messages to the right muscles to get started and keep going, and your feet take turns doing their job. And at the same time, you are watching for sidewalk irregularities and other obstacles. Your vast nerve network, from head to toe, is magnificent, to say the least. A vast number of operations are happening concurrently. And we take it all for granted. We need to continually tune up our nervous system to be ready for those emergencies that will, for sure, come sooner or later.

Please walk where it's safe. Well lighted, smooth firm surfaces, allow you to concentrate on walking safely. Some people are very awkward when they walk because their arms and legs are not coordinated for the best walking action. The correct action for walking is when the left foot is forward the right arm is also forward, and vice versa.

This opposite upper-body and lower-body action counterbalances the twist of the hip position as you walk. Walking in place, in this manner, is called Cross Crawl. The arms are vigorously pumping as the knees are raised higher than usual with each step. A good workout is guaranteed right in your living room when you merely Cross Crawl. You become a parade of one marching to some music. J.P. Sousa will be glad to join you.

There are many walking variations. Each obliges the brain to respond by solving novel motor problems. It is this demand that beautifully stimulates the brain and makes it better.

We must immediately respond to a stumble. Apathy and/or disease can quickly erode your response speed. Under these conditions, the nervous system will not function up to par. You need to be ready for possible emergencies. The body is marvelously malleable and can accommodate extensive remediation. It will get better if and when you consistently work it. You never know how much better you can become until you try.

Note: All KAT tools stimulate the brain in different ways. If you try them all, no part of the brain and body is left out. Practice by opening the exercise door and you will:

move out . . . move on . . . move up.

Walking Variations

-Walk straight, using a floor line as your guide -- perfect for anti-wobble practice
-As you walk, look farther ahead but still see your toes with peripheral vision
-Walk in place with your eyes closed; hold on to a door jam if needed
-Walk first with your legs wide apart, then close together, as on a tight rope
-Walk with first one hand and then both hands over your head, and then clasp your hands behind your back as you walk
-Take bigger steps -- even a small increase in step length will improve balance
-Walk duck-footed, then pigeon-toed
-Walk heavy, walk light
-Walk a zigzag walk
-Walk fast, then slow, then normally
-Walk first flat-footed, then on your toes
-Walk on your heels, then on your toes
-Walk sideways, but be careful of tripping on your own feet as they cross
-Walk as if on ice
-Walk as if sneaking up on your teen-aged friend
-Walk as if you are depressed and dejected, then as if you are joyful and happy
-Walk heavy-footed, now light-footed
-Walk with your knees bent; then walk stiff-legged
- Walk tall -- walk small
- Walk as you hum a tune
- Rhythmically count steps by ones or twos, and then count backward from a large number
- Match your footfalls to the meter of a poem or song
- Breathe to the cadence of your footfalls
- As you walk, look for things nearby, then things far away
- Walk looking left, then right, using your eyes only. Then move your head right to left in rhythm with your footfalls
- Do the elephant walk; i.e., lumber with your "trunk" (arms) swinging
- Dance by yourself or with another person
- With every other footfall, focus on a different object. Use peripheral vision to locate the next object before you look at it directly
- Sing as you walk in rhythm with your footfalls
- Walk with one foot a little lighter than the other, in a kind of limp
- Walk with excellent posture
- Decide to step on each sidewalk crack, and then refuse to step on any lines. (Notice that you must vary your gait)
- Become aware of walking rhythms, and then add talking cadences
- Walk while tossing a ball from hand to hand in time with footfalls
- Breathe in for four paces, and then out for four paces, varying your breathing cadence
- Walk slowly with a book or beanbag, or one sheet of toilet paper on your head
- Whistle while you walk to the rhythm of your footfalls
- Count forward or backwards, or say the alphabet with each footfall or every other footfall. Count forward, backward, count by twos or more. Count in a foreign language. Count with nonsense sounds but as you count, think of the orthodox number

- One walking variation that should be performed more than one time a day is to take *longer, larger steps than normal.* (See the segments entitled, Longer, Larger Steps and Line and Spot Walking

Direct Vision and Peripheral Vision

Direct vision is how you see what you look at while peripheral vision is what you see with your side vision. Both direct and peripheral vision are vital for good balance.

You may practice your peripheral vision many times a day. A specific exercise is to focus directly on your stretched hand in front of your eyes. At the same time, purposefully become peripherally aware of what is beyond and to the left and right of your hand. This is peripheral vision. Then reverse the task by focusing beyond your hand, but purposefully "see" your hand via peripheral vision.

Peripheral vision can also be exercised while walking. Young people walk with little conscious visual attention to their feet. Their peripheral vision is doing the job of helping them avoid pitfalls. But as we age and/or become disabled and, as our visual abilities diminish, we are duty-bound to practice attentively so our visual abilities remain as sharp as possible. Practice does make a difference.

Try this. As you walk, focus directly on the ground about 10 to 20 feet in front of you. At the same time, focus your peripheral attention on your feet. You will be aware of your feet coming in view with each step. As this becomes easier, focus farther and farther in front of yourself while retaining awareness on your feet with your peripheral vision. If you focus too far ahead, your feet can't be seen. With practice you will be make this skill more automatic and thus improve your walking safety.

The subtle part of this exercise is that as you focus afar, your peripheral vision, along with accompanying attention, is aiding your decision-making process on just where to step next. This unconscious decision making ability also diminishes with age and disability. Practice will help keep you better balanced over your feet. At first, if this practice does not feel safe for you, begin by walking in place.

One more exercise. Walk while slowly moving your head from side to side. Begin with small movements at first, and then progress to swiveling from side to side as far as you can go, all while walking. Again, you might begin while walking in place and/or holding onto a support.

You will find that tool manipulation is better achieved with good use of the eyes. Repetitious practice renders even poor eyes more efficient. Eye-hand and eye-foot coordination is the goal.

Finger Pointing and Attention Switching

In Attention Switching, you exercise conscious control over the direction and use of your eyes. Each of the six very small control muscles in each eye requires exercise, as well as the mind's ability to decide where to look. Also, Attention Switching enhances your ability to attend.

Attention switching can be done either sitting or standing. Sitting may feel safer, but standing will add the challenge of maintaining balance. Direct your eyes across the room to an object or a structural feature. Restrict your gaze to that one point. Concentrate on that point for about two counts. During this time interval, your peripheral vision locates the next looking point. Then quickly move your gaze to the new point. Try this slowly at first. Perform Attention Switching several times a day till it becomes accurate and easy. By the way, the longer you can do any repetitive act at one session, the more you have bettered your ability to attend to your own personal goals. Always perform in a regular cadence, i.e. to a musical beat or a metronome, or, merely count out your own rhythm. It is ok to walk in rhythm to the pace of your repetitive refocusing. One step per visual change is good. Also, some students like to point while they perform Attention Switching. Try it with or without pointing.

Longer, Steps (LS)

After a fall or hospital stay, you may become fearful of moving as you once did. Frequently, the outcome of this fear is smaller and smaller steps. Yes, smaller steps do make walking more stable, but in the long run smaller steps can be counter productive to safe locomotion. Why? Small steps soon leave hip and leg muscles shortened. This lack of flexibility makes it difficult or impossible to step over a pothole or react to balance emergencies. Also, taking short steps slows you down, we come to think we are old, and we stay longer and longer on the couch. A sedentary life style makes everything worse. Short strides are the path to great instability. The answer is to purposefully practice enlarging your steps as much as possible. Longer steps can be done safely.

Research has shown that purposefully practicing longer steps than normal helps people to recover more quickly from stumbles. Taking larger steps keeps hip joints more flexible, strengthens ankles and legs, and enhances coordination between the upper and lower body. Longer steps also allow faster walking. Longer steps require more balance time between each step. In fact, walking is a series of one-leg balances.

Try this. When you walk down a hallway, in the mall, or around the block, mark off a specified distance such as between two doorways, or the distance between two telephone poles. Then walk that distance in your normal manner, counting each step. Remember that number. Now walk the same distance and try to reduce the number of steps. Fewer strides mean longer steps. And longer steps, even if they are just a tiny bit more than usual, challenge the balance mechanisms in your body and brain. With practice, you will be able to take longer steps even better if you stretch your leg and hip muscles. Stiff muscles are one cause of the shuffling gait that no one wants. Vigorously pumping your arms assists in taking longer steps. Arm action is more important to sound walking than most of us think.

Purposefully practicing longer steps is a simple activity, requiring no equipment, or professional trainer. You become your own trainer. All you need is yourself saying, like the little engine that could, I can too. You merely need to increase your stride length a little bit at a time today, then a little more tomorrow. If even a little change in your stride is frightening, slide your hand along a wall for support as you practice. You will be surprised how much true confidence this simple support will provide. Under these conditions, you can concentrate on taking longer steps.

Here is the true story of a man whose back condition precluded him from ever walking without the walker. Even with the walker he took small and labored steps. But we found a way for him to fully participate in class activities. He stood wedged in a corner, which freed both his hands to handle KAT tools. He also was asked to take longer steps during the day. After six weeks of class, he said his greatest achievement was that now he could walk faster. That meant he was habitually taking longer steps. Walking even a little faster is no small accomplishment for a man who thought he could never improve. It was obvious his well-being was enhanced. He was now less hesitant about going to events because he could get there with greater satisfaction.

Line and Spot-Walking

No one, whether young or old, blind or sighted, ever walks in a perfectly straight line. However, under some conditions, wobbling becomes dangerous. Walking in relation to lines is a good anti-wobble exercise.

Begin simply by walking with one foot stepping a line on the floor and the other off the line. The line is an unwavering guide for staying straight. Walk with good posture and look to the front with your peripheral vision seeing your feet. If you step off the line, don't worry; just get back on with the next step. Soon you'll get the hang of it.

Then advance to walking as if on a tight rope, with one foot following the other on the line on the floor. Perhaps you can only do this for two or three steps. Keep trying; you will get better at it. If tight rope walking is too much for you begin by holding on to someone, or use a cane. Safety is of prime concern.

Line walking can be done anywhere you find a line. Most malls have tile floors. The edges of the tiles are good lines to use. In your home, you could put down a masking tape line and walk along it, while using a wall for support. Look for lines in your world and you will find them.

Now you can try the opposite of line walking. You can walk adjacent to the line, and then step back and forth over it in a rhythmic pattern. Many walking patterns involve the use of lines. Invent some for yourself. An example, purposeful zigzagging is balance control.

As you progress in line-walking you will build endurance. Slowly advance your walking goals: line-walk for a designated distance, and then next week, walk farther on the line. Many people find they can walk farther when their mind and body are engaged with balance challenges. Concentrated learning knocks boredom cold.

Keep in mind that all learning should be sequenced from simple actions to activities that are more complex. Begin with small, short-term goals. They will add up to noticeable improvements.

Now consider *spot walking*. Remember that old saying, "If you step on a crack you'll break your mother's back"? (Not true, of course. It is a frightening thing to tell children.) Cracks in the sidewalk and spots on the floor can become useful balance tools. As you walk your daily rounds, become aware of the many blemishes, blotches, cracks, discoloration, dots, lines, marks, smudges, specks, splotches, spots, stains, and especially potholes in and on your walking surfaces. Visually choose a spot ahead of you. Make a conscious decision to step on it, or avoid it, as you walk. If someone asks what are you doing, tell him or her you have invented a new form of hopscotch. Get them to try it, and explain why it is good. They will benefit too.

Many malls have floors with different color blocks of tile. As you approach a different color block, determine to step on a certain block with, say, your left foot. To do this you must adjust your gait in length, speed, and direction. The length, speed, and direction of your gait must be kept under conscious control. As you walk, continually search for the next spot to step on. You are looking, deciding, and stepping all at the same time. Doing more than one thing at a time is a wonderful challenge to the nervous system. All this takes attention, which is also heightened, by spot walking.

For fun KAT calls this exercise PHAP: *Pot Hole Avoidance Practice*. PHAP requires that you maintain and continually enhance your ability to avoid a wobble or slip, a stagger or lurch, a stumble or trip. PHAP will also strengthen your ability to attend to your walking.

Line and spot walking will enhance your ability to react positively to emergencies. And emergencies can and will come. Be ready. A dubious older gentleman in my class said, "I'll try spot walking, but just in case this doesn't help my balance, I will at least know all the spots and lines around my block." Now that's a positive attitude. He did try it. Reporting back, he said he could now walk faster, longer, and safer. He reflected that he now looks forward to his walk because he is more confident, and his walk time seems to fly.

Life presents many potholes. There are going to be problems, but if you are prepared, you are in control. And you do have much untapped controlling power. Strengthen your capacities with practice, which is initiated by your will. Make a regular time to practice. Practice with a friend is productive. When you try hard at anything the Marines will honor you for becoming: *The best you can be.*

How does walking lines and spot walking help your balance? Your brain and eyes are a long way from your feet. When you use lines and spots in your walking you are making conscious decisions about where to put your feet. In so doing, you strengthen the connection between your brain, eyes and feet. Here's an obvious statement:

When you place your feet in the right place
at the right time, all the time, you will never fall.

Attention to the lines and spots will help you achieve better reaction time and adjustment ability.

The next section on Tandem Walking is similar to Line Walking. However, Tandem Walking is a bit more advanced.

Tandem Walking (TW) (Tight Roping)

Tandem walking is the name for walking a floor line as if on a tightrope. One foot is placed directly in front of the other as you walk. But obviously there is little danger because the line is flat on the floor. However, if your balance is precarious, hang onto a treadmill handrail or a railing. You may also walk parallel to a wall with one hand sliding along for support. Of course, another person may give you support.

Walk slowly at first. Concentrate on how each foot must step directly in front of the other. Use your eyes to check your foot placement. If things are going well, look straight ahead, while paying particular attention to your peripheral vision to guide the placement of your feet. Great somatosensory enhancement occurs when walking with your eyes closed, holding onto a railing, or sliding your hand along. Safe blind walking forces the nerves all over your body to become responsible for what the eyes usually do.

Ordinary walking is, of course, more secure than tandem walking because the narrow foot placement eliminates much of the lateral ground support. The value of challenging the nervous system with TW is to force internal solutions to the balance problem. In a sense, the nervous system is forced to learn a new and complicated neurological dance. The somatosensory and visual balance systems are tested by this new motor challenge. Your goal is to generate new brain/body neurological connections by working toward your goal in a safe and prudent manner.

> Note: The term somatosensory may be confusing. Soma means body and sensory refers to the nerves which receive information, especially from the joints and skin. There are three balance control systems. The Balance Control Systems section details the action and interrelationships of the somatosensory, the vision and the vestibular systems. It is good to know how your body works.

To the Rear March

Walking skills include turning to the left, right, and all the way around. Turning is sometimes precarious. We can practice as an Army drill sergeant would direct us.

First, the goal is to turn to the left. Walk slowly forward. When your right foot reaches the place you wish to turn, plant your right foot solidly on the ground, pointed about 45 degrees to the left. Pivot on it to make a one-quarter turn, (90 degrees), to the left, then step out in the new direction with your left foot. The Army calls this *to the left march.* Reverse the directions and go to the right.

To The Rear March is much the same as above, but demands a one-half turn, which sends you back the way you came. Follow the above direction but this time pivot all the way back 180 degrees. If your balance is unsteady, do not try this without a helper.

> Note: At the end of this chapter you will notice that *To The Rear March* will come in handy with the test called Get Up and Go.

Laser Walking (LW)

Laser Walking (LW) is an exciting, new brain/body exercise. Laser Walking requires all three-brain integration dimensions to become simultaneously active. For emphasis, I repeat the three-dimensional avenues of the brain: *cross-brain lobe reciprocality* = communication, *front-to-back* = focus; and *top-to-bottom* = centering. Of course, neural commutation goes both ways in each of the three dimensions.

Please perform the following direction in order, one through four.
Part one: Preparatory for LW. Sit in a chair. As you lift your right leg off the ground, touch your right thigh with your left hand. Now lift the left leg and touch it with your right hand. Repeat. Brain Gym, a neurologically based set of exercises and postures, calls this Cross Crawl. Now stand and do the Cross Crawl. Try not to bend down, but rather keep your upright posture by bringing your knees up high. If this is precarious, stand with your back to a wall or stand in the corner.

Part two: Sit in a chair. Lift your right leg off the ground as above, but this time instead of touching your right thigh with your left hand, aim your left forefinger toward your right foot. As your shoe touches the floor, as in walking, imagine a very short burst of soft laser light coming from your left forefinger and instantly hitting your right foot. Now do the same on the other side, with your right index finger shooting the laser beam hitting the left foot. Slowly alternate till you get all four limbs working smoothly together, each time hitting the foot with your imaginary laser beam.

Part three: Now stand with your left hand out in front with your right foot also out in front. Connect the two with a burst of laser light. Now try the other side. Do this until you are comfortable with the coordination of all four limbs. You are merely walking in place, but with bursts of timed laser light between hands and feet.

Part four: Now try it as you walk slowly. Attempt to fire the laser bursts at the instant your foot hits the floor. Some like to imagine that their beam is brightly colored. One man told me he would use the colors of the rainbow–*yellow, orange, red, green, blue, purple and indigo*–in their proper sequence. Then he repeated the sequence, but now backwards. This is a great mental-motor coordination activity. Also, Laser Walking demands the upper body and the lower body work together, which is the same demand when we walk. Later you can perform laser finger pointing by using each of the five fingers in order.

Laser Walking encourages functional coordination between your hands and feet. Also benefited, is the coordination between the two lobes of the brain. Laser walking is a marvelous example of cross lateral communication, as well as concurrence, which is doing more than one thing at a time. The goal is to keep your mind so busy with attention-developing accomplishments that you retain your ability to concentrate into old age. The *use-it-or-lose-it* principle comes into play here because both the brain and the body, i.e., the nerves and the muscles, are being harmonized in a series of coordinated actions.

Lazy 8

The Lazy 8 is also a very good Brain Gym eye/hand exercise for balance. In addition, it will prepare you for Infinity Walking, described next. The Lazy 8 is a rudimentary exercise and is similar to the V warm up exercise of KAT's Kai Bhi exercise form.

Begin the Lazy 8 with either hand at least 14 inches in front of your face. Focus on your Thumb nail. You draw an 8 on its side, (∞) which is an infinity sign. Always begin from the middle of the ∞, tracing in the air toward the upper left, looping to the left half of the ∞, then around the ∞, coming back to the middle. Without stopping, continue on to the upper right and back around to your beginning position. Repeat at least ten complete lazy eights. Perform with both hands separately, and then both hands together.

Make it more of a whole body exercise by rocking from side to side, as you draw. Do your best to keep the left and right circles the same size. Draw your lazy 8 as big as the arms will reach. Bend your knees on the lower part of the 8 and up on your toes on the high side of the 8.

Make it harder by separating the two hands about four inches. Allow the left hand to lead as the right follows in the lazy 8 pattern. Try to keep the hands the same distance apart and on exactly the same path. This will challenge your concentration. Accuracy comes with practice. The two lobes of the brain must work together to perform this move. Greater and greater brain integration is the goal.

The Brain Gym version of the Lazy 8 is done with focus on the thumb. The KAT version, called Kai Bhi, adds a small object that becomes a focal point as it is transferred from hand to hand in coordination with the lazy eight pattern. Your visual focus should be on the ball. When one movement cycle is completed, the ball (or any object) may be transferred to the other hand as it repeats the Lazy 8 pattern.

Infinity Walking (IW)

In brief, Infinity Walking asks you to walk in a figure 8 pattern. First, stand and imagine a large 8 on the floor in front of you. Begin walking to the left of the lower loop of the 8. Walk directly across the middle and continue to the upper circle of the 8 and back to the starting point. Keep going at least 10 times around. Walking the 8 pattern is the same as drawing an 8, only beginning and ending on the bottom.

To better keep track of where you are in the eight pattern, you might place a chair in the middle of each of the loops of the 8 pattern. After some practice, you perform the Infinity Walking pattern from memory.

The turns of a figure 8 demand first a clockwise turn, and then a counterclockwise turn. When walking the eight pattern becomes more automatic, you are asked to combine walking with other motor skills and activities. Some of these activities include conversing with others, telling stories, reciting poetry, calculating simple arithmetic problems, counting backwards from a hundred, or continually turning your head toward one wall as you walk the 8. I interpret the purpose of Infinity Walking as being similar to Kinetic Arts Training's basic purpose. In both, the body, through its movement, stimulates and integrates the brain, leading to an outcome of more intricate (functional) neural patterns. At the same time, the body becomes more graceful and balanced.

One prime feature of Infinity Walking is the fact that each time you turn right or left, your brain hemispheres switches dominance. Thus, the two lobes are making their inter-communication more precise. Brain efficiency is part of good balance.

If you would like to find out more, read *Infinity Walk: Book 1– The Physical Self*, by Deborah Sunbeck, Ph.D. See www.infinitywalk.com Dr. Sunbeck's books are informative, provocative, and offer practical ideas to improve your balance.

Inclined Plane

Negotiating stairs is a problem for some. Even more precarious, for some, is walking up or down a hill, like the wheelchair entrance ramp. Remember, your ankles are the first line of defense against falls. But your ankles (along with the rest of you) are habituated to the horizontal surfaces. A tilted surface can cause confusion. The ankles need to keep their ability to make quick adjustments so that we can negotiate tilts, slants, slopes and inclines. Walking practice on an inclined plane or on hills will help keep you safe and your balance in high maintenance. If there is a choice of stair or a handicapped entrance, occasionally choose the inclined plane, even if you do not think you need it. When you walk around the block, don't curse the hills; take their challenge as a balance lesson.

Obstacle Curse

Many people think of the world as an obstacle curse, rather than a course. Here's some advice. Simplify the traffic patterns in your home. Sometimes we do forget what is where and fall over even familiar things. Light all areas well. Make all possible improvements so you can honestly say that you have done all you can to make your home safe. Better to be safe than cursing from a hospital bed.

Combining balance exercises with a homemade obstacle course is good. For instance, purposely walk all the way around a chair, just for practice. The skill of avoiding obstacles requires vision as well as a coordinated body. Seeing where to place your next footfall and avoiding what is dangerous means you know just where you are in space. Balance requires continually accurate spatial adjustment.

Spot Walking as suggested above will improve this skill. Life's obstacles, whether emotional or physical act as a challenge to become stronger and more alert. They can stimulate your ability to grow or you could interpret them as a curse. Your choice.

Standing Wall Tall

Old or young, we all need to be reminded what vertical is. Good posture is a powerful factor in good balance. Stand tall with your buttocks, shoulder blades, and head touching the wall. Stretch tall, pull in your middle, and then slowly walk away retaining your erect posture.

A wall is a reliable reminder to stand and walk Vertical. Upright is good. However, remember that the small of the back is meant to curve inward so it will not remain touching the wall for long. Even a few Wall Tall practices a day will strengthen your back muscles. Standing and walking is a fight with gravity. Independent life is when you win the struggle.

Stretching up against gravity is a kind of weight-lifting exercise. Standing tall will not make you uppity. Wall Tall practice makes good posture a habit. People will notice.

After a couple of experiences with walking wall tall, I ask the question, what do a scarf, a handkerchief, a beanbag, or a single sheet of toilet paper have in common? Answer: All are light and soft, which makes them just right to put on top of your head. Purpose? I've discovered that when people walk tall with an object on their heads, they are challenged to retain their good posture longer. The strategy is to walk slowly and smoothly for progressively longer periods. One sheet of toilet paper on the head is the lightest object and therefore the hardest to work with, but it is by far the most fun.

Any object on your head is a simple reminder of your purpose. Would-be models learn to walk tall and lithe by walking with a book on their head. Good posture is a large factor in solid balance and general health. (After walking tall for a couple of weeks, you will most likely be asked to pose for the cover of a national fitness magazine. But don't feel obliged to bare your navel . . . unless of course they offer you a belly-button bonus.)

The Greene Wall Lean

This is a standing wall tall variation suggested by Bob Greene, a famous physical trainer.

Begin as above, standing with your back and head touching the wall. Now inch your feet, buttocks, and spine away from the wall while your head remains learning on the wall. Even a little slant puts you in the Greene Wall Lean. The body remains as straight as if you were standing vertically. Greene suggests 30 seconds, but I suggest that at first you do it just as long as you are comfortable. As you become stronger, you will lean longer. Again, always be safe.

The Greene Wall Lean is a back-strengthening exercise. A strong back is required for good posture and stable balance. As you progress, your feet will move farther and farther away from the wall. Let your arms hang vertically and relax. The goal is to keep your body straight even while in the leaning position.

What happens in this exercise? As you stand exaggeratedly tall next to the wall, you are in a very strange position that is much different from normal. When you do the Greene Lean you are not only standing tall but also you must increase the muscle tone in your back in order to keep leaning. When you put effort into the lean and walk away tall, you have told your back muscles, in no uncertain terms, which position you want to maintain good posture. Of course, as always, I plead with you to *Do what you can, then just a little bit more.* Also, don't try to walk in this extra tall position too long at first. As time goes on you can increase the *duration* (time) spent in the leaning position. In other words, throughout your day, do the Greene Wall Lean *frequently*. The *intensity* of the exercise increases with the distance your feet are from the wall. *Duration, frequency, and intensity* are the three ways to manipulate the effort you put into your workouts.

Upright posture is worth considerable effort to change. Then soon:

You'll look like a tall and willowy bean
as you angle your stance in the Greene Wall Lean.
Stiffen your back, then walk away.
After a while it's all child's play.

Your friends will wonder what you have done.
You smile more now, life is more fun.
So kudos to Greene we love ya' a lot,
cause when we stand tall we ain't got no pot.

One-Leg Balance

Hold on to the doorjamb, chair back, or wall for support. Raise one leg and stabilize it by gently placing the raised foot on the lower calf of the standing leg. Focus your eyes on a spot on the floor about 10 to 15 feet in front. Become aware of your body, especially the alignment of your hips and shoulder over your ankles. When satisfied that you are erect, then let go of your support. Return to the wall whenever you wish. Practice repeatedly. Focused attention will speed your balance skill enhancement. You will gradually be able to stand on one leg for longer periods. Practice a few times a day for best results. Short practice sessions are best.

One-leg balance can be done performing daily tasks. For instance, while at the kitchen counter, stand on one leg for a short time, and not always on the same leg. It's ok if one hip is touching the wall when you begin. Standing on one leg in this way will help to renew leg and hip strength that you might have lost. Ankle rotation exercises are good for strengthening ankles and resistance training will strengthen the muscles in the entire leg. Remember, the ankles are your first line of defense against falls. See the section on the three defenses against falls found in the previous Knowledge chapter. Make it all a game and enjoy the success that follows.

Many people have asked me why they can perform a one-leg balance when just one finger is touching the wall. My response is that their somatosensory system is still in great working order. Your finger on the wall tells you what vertical is, and gives you a feeling of safe support. This all happens through the somatosensory system. It is the vast network of nerves feeding the brain with information from every muscle fiber, joint and the entire skin's surface. It tells you where you are in space and what to do to keep balanced. The other two systems that control balance are the vestibular system (inner ear) and vision. One-leg balance principally activates the somatosensory and the visual balance systems.

Walking is merely a rhythmic series of one-leg balances. When you walk, you step from the left foot to the right, then right to the left, etc. While one foot is in the air coming forward for the next step, you are balanced on one leg. Standing quietly on one leg is harder than when shifting from foot to foot when walking. But there is great value in the practice. One-leg balance will strengthen your legs, as you challenge your nervous system to perform more securely.

If you wish to measure the progress of your one-leg balance, measure in seconds the length of time balancing on one leg. You can approximate your time by counting, one thousand one, etc. If you have a metronome, you can count the seconds more accurately. Or a friend can time you with a stopwatch. The main thing is to love the journey from now to better. Reminder: You are the vehicle.

It's a lotta fun to stand on just one.
You'll enjoy your success more than a ton.
You can do it better when you practice right.
And soon your joy will be high like a kite.

The one-leg balance record is held by a Sri Lankan man. So says *The Guinness Book of World Records*. In May of 1997, he stood on one leg for 76 hours and 40 minutes. Personally, I do not wish to compete with anyone. However, our own optimum physiological balance is the record we should all shoot for. When you push just a little each day, better is waiting to embrace you.

Wall Kicking

Here's an obvious statement:

When you place your feet in the right place,
at the right time,
all the time,
you will never fall.

The goal is to keep your center of gravity within the your limits of balance ability. The trick is to find safe practice procedures to achieve the goal. Wall Kicking is a safe activity. Stand facing a wall with your feet about six inches away from the wall. Gaining support from the wall, tap the wall lightly with one toe, then with the other. Soon you will be able to consistently tap the wall with uniform pressure and do so in a regular rhythm.

Here are some variations:
-Try Wall Kicking with your eyes closed
- Vary your distance from the wall
- Stand with your back against the wall, and reach back and kick the wall with your heels
- Kick in patterns, such as two kicks with the left foot and one with the right, etc
- Lengthen the exercise by tapping to the beat of music. Make an effort to perform this activity for a whole song. If you are tired when finished, sit, lie, nap, whatever, but be proud you are pushing yourself to become more able than you were before
- More advanced is wall kicking without holding onto wall, and with eyes closed
- When you kick the wall with your foot do the same with your hand on the same side
- Make your hand and foot touch at exactly the same instant. (Again, notice the concept of concurrency.)
- As you face the wall, imagine that your feet are placed on a clock face, with your left foot on 9 and the right on 3. Begin with the right foot. Kick the wall and when it returns place it on 4. When the left foot returns, place it at the 10, and so forth around the clock face.

You will soon notice that you must turn all the way around to cover the clock face. Also, notice that there are ways to support yourself on the wall no matter which direction you are facing.

Wall kicking, whether simple or complex, requires movement, placement, sequence, planning, memory, and timing. All these need to be handled neurologically. Even holding onto the wall, as you rotate, is a problem to be worked out. We never learn anything in an instant. Discouragement is not an option. The skill will come; stay with it. The brain loves the trial and error process. Discover your own way to perform the wall-kicking dance. Success feels good because well-deserved pride adds zest to life.

Dance

Someone wrote, *Life may not be the party we hoped for, but while we are here, we might as well dance.* Dance to your favorite music. The emotion connected to joyful movement is very healthy. You can't be uptight and dance well. Loose-like-a-goose is good. Focus on the beat and stay with it. When you can't find a partner, find a line-dance or square dance group. When you're alone, really let yourself go. Dancing can loosen up those stiff parts in you.

Become a kid again and dance to Swing, do the Cha-Cha, or how about the Twist. Whatever your high school favorite dance was, do it and remember those good times. Mental regression along with appropriate rhythmic physical movement is a health push toward more youthful vigor.

Baton

Make a durable, well-weighted baton using a stack of 8 to 10 full-sized sheets of newspaper. Position them so you can read the paper. Make a half-inch fold on the bottom edge of the stack nearest you. Now roll using both hands. Two persons rolling the same baton is best. Make the roll as tight and even as possible. When you are finished, wrap a few strips of tape around it and you will have a 23 inch baton.

First, place the baton in one hand and exchange it to the other behind your back. Keep it going in one direction, then reverse. Listen to the sound of the baton slapping your hand as you make the exchange. Vary the intensity of the slap.

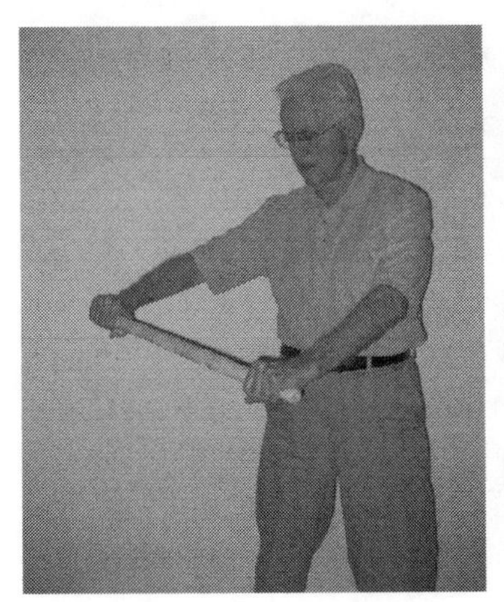

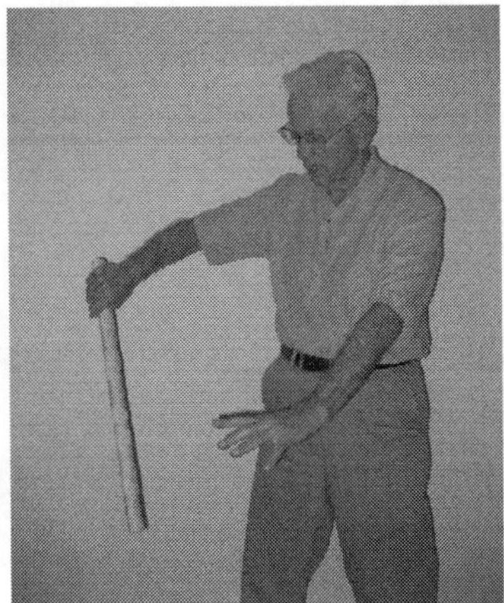

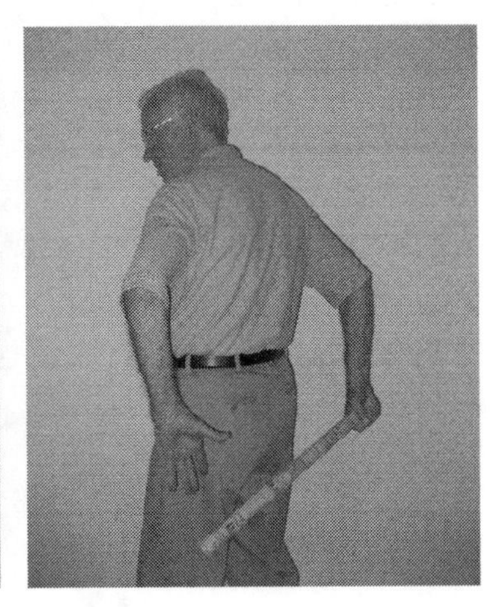

Another variation is to place the baton in your right hand. Lift your right leg and bend at the knee. Transfer the baton under your right leg to your left hand. Then lift the left leg and pass the baton under it. When you want an aerobic workout, repeat the action keeping your body erect and lifting your legs as high as possible. For a stronger heart, keep it up till you are a bit winded. Lungs also become strong when exercised. Keep at it day after day and your aerobic conditioning will improve. Breathing hard gets rid of all that old and stale couch potato air. Music helps to increase your stick-to-a-tive-ness.

Hold the baton in its middle with one hand then toss in the air just an inch or so. Try the other hand. Now toss it from hand to hand. Now turn your hand over and drop and catch the baton as in Crabbing. Almost anything you can do with a ball can be done with a baton.

Hold the baton in one hand with the palm up. Look at the other end, then flip it so it makes a half rotation in the air, and catch it on the other end, still with the palm up. At first toss it and catch it with the same hand. Then flip it from hand to hand. Short practices sessions are best. Keep your baton handy so you can practice several times a day. Show off your skill to others who will soon recognize that they too are still able to learn new skills. And with every bit of success, praise yourself. Go ahead, you earned it.

Now flip the baton a full rotation in the air, which allows you to catch it on the same end from which it was tossed. Concentrate on your visual ability to see the baton spin in the air and anticipate just where to catch it in its rotation.

Any elongated object can become a baton, such as a pencil or a spoon. Each item has its own airborne gyrational dynamics. It is fascinating to see and feel the difference among various items. If you find you enjoy this, you might be considered as crazy as most jugglers. (Perhaps "passionate" is the more diplomatic term).

To show you that I am serious about practice I offer the following Rap:

Work like a Devil, then let up a bit.
Never never feel like an idi-it.
Practice and practice as much as you're able.
Then do something good
like contemplate your navel.

Horizontal Yardstick or Baton Balancing

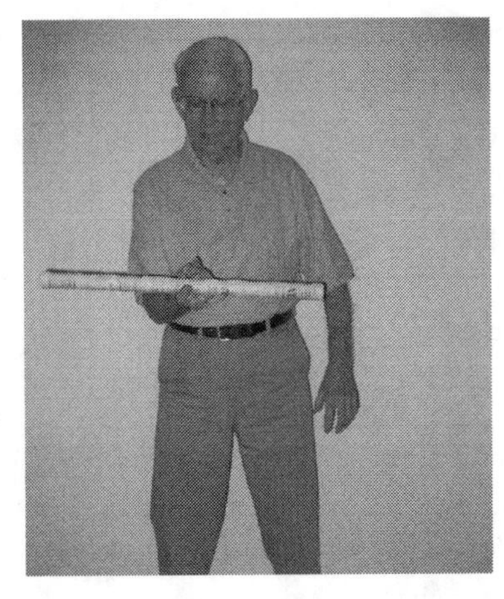

Begin with a yardstick or any stick at least 2 feet long. By sight and feel, find the middle of the object and balance it horizontally on your four, palm-up fingers, then on three, then two, then on one finger. Make it harder by walking and moving the stick from side to side and/or up and down. Try it with your eyes closed. Try balancing two sticks, one on each hand and fingers. Horizontal balancing is good preparation for the vertical balancing of a cone.

Cone Balancing

The best object for balancing I know is simply made from two or three sheets of ordinary newspaper. Lay them out flat on a table. Place them so they can be read. If you are right-handed, begin by folding the right lower corner inward about four inches. Make a sharp crease. Now with your right hand on the right lower corner, begin to tightly roll the paper upward, while your left hand loosely guides the rolling process. Your right hand must keep the roll compact while your left allows the larger part of the cone to form. Continue rolling till you have a cone. When you are finished, the top of the cone should be between two and three inches in diameter. Prepare a small bit of tape ahead of time to put on the middle of the cone to hold it in shape. The small end is the bottom of the cone. You have achieved your goal of fashioning a cheap, safe and efficient cone for balancing practice. (For those who are impaired, a good preparation for cone balancing is to use a yardstick and balance it horizontally as suggested in the previous section.)

Begin your cone-balancing practice in an unoccupied corner of the room. Place the pointed end of the cone between the pads of your index and third finger. The cone's flared end leans into the corner. Now slowly move your fingertips toward the corner. Soon the top of the cone will come off the wall. Quickly jerk your hand back toward yourself and the top of the cone will fall back into the corner. This action will activate a quick reaction. Response speed is necessary in case of emergencies. Mastering this, go on to the next level.

The cone is a great gift for children. As grandparents, my wife and I began a Christmas cone ritual. On the Christmas tree, there appears a paper cone for everyone in the family. We began this tradition on our first grandchild's first Christmas. Of course, he could not balance a cone at less than one year of age. But all our grandchildren now see us performing cone balancing at least once a year. We will do this every year and when their nervous systems are ready, they will join the activity. It will be 'the thing to do' as part of Christmas morning.

From the standpoint of child development, as well as gerontology, cone balancing is highly valuable. The challenge heightens curiosity, expectation of success is triggered, and motor experimentalism is stimulated. Human neurology, regardless of age, demands a challenge to maintain and improve its function.

Rope

Allow a rope, about three and a half feet long, to hang down loosely from your fingertips. Begin to make circular movements with your arm, wrist and fingers. When you find the right rotational speed, the rope will form a C shape. Perform this in both a clockwise and counterclockwise movement. Try it with your other hand.

Rope Variations

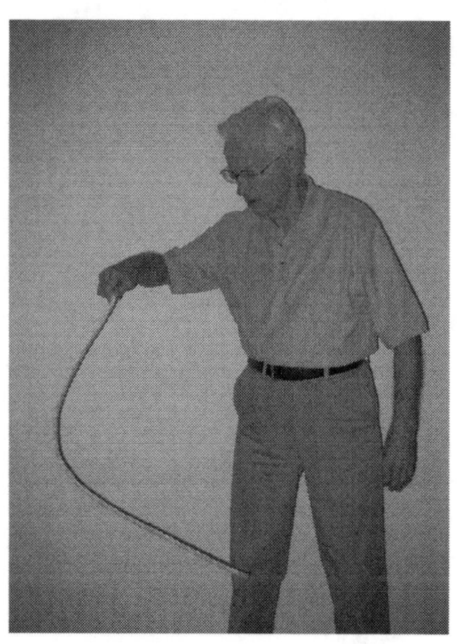

- See if you can retain the C shape with your eyes closed. Even if your first attempt fails, you will soon become more sensitive to the feel of the rope
- With a rope in each hand, make two Cs at the same time.
- Hold the rope with your fingertips on one end. Quickly jerk the rope straight up, let go, and then catch it on the other end with the same hand. Now try tossing it up with one hand then catching it on the other end with the other hand. Hint: It helps to keep the rope as straight and as vertical as possible.
- Hold the rope out to one side. Then swing the rope over your head. Now grab the other end with your other hand, Repeat back and forth up over your head. Keep your eyes on the rope.
- Start by holding the end of the rope on the right side of your body. Swing the rope in one circle, and then quickly change sides with one circle on the left side. Continue back and forth. This action forms a 3 D figure eight pattern.
- Whip the rope in a circular motion so that you hear "the wind in its sail," so to speak.

Note: With all KAT tools, you are encouraged to perform each activity in an ever-smoother more efficient fashion. Practice in a variety of positions, such as standing, leaning against a wall, seated, eyes shut, while standing on one leg, or reciting a poem . . . you get the idea. Variety is good for brain growth. You will become a better problem solver by challenging yourself with more and harder problems.

Knot Tying

There is no end to the number of knots that can be learned. For instance, *The Ashley Book of Knots* describes 3,900 knots. Each one is different, and some are more challenging than others. To take another example, macramé is a beautiful demonstration of knot-tying possibilities.

Why is knot tying good for balance? Any exercise that requires the body to visually and physically control right from left, over from under, and near from far, as well as perform each move in an exact sequence is good for the brain and body. Knot tying connects the four dimensions of the outside world, (north, east, south, and west), to the four dimensions of the brain (focus, communication, centering, and timing (rhythm).

Brush up on the knots you already know how to tie. I love a square knot because its beautiful symmetry which is a good metaphor for balance. The square knot requires simple two-handed cooperation. It is easiest to learn the square knot if you have a rope in hand while reading the directions. The rope or thick string can be about two or more feet long. Simply, it is *left over right and right over left.* Here's more details. Hold the two ends of the rope, one end in each hand, so the ends are pointing toward the ceiling. Now bring the two together and hold both in the right hand. About five inches or so of rope ends are between your holding hand and the ends. Now the left hand moves the left rope end over the right end. It is then tucked under. This is half the knot. The right end is then moved over the left end. Leave enough rope to complete the second sequence. Now place the right end over the left and tuck it through. Remembering the sequence *of left over right, right over left*, helps you to remember the correct sequence. A granny knot occurs when you repeat left over right at both stages of tying. The granny knot is dramatically different from the real square knot.

Knot tying is a process that contains a number of steps. For me, the square knot has six steps. It may be different for you. Counting seems to facilitate memory of sequence. Experiment and come out with the right number of counting steps for you. When you can tie the knot easily, synchronize each footfall with each tying step. Practice till you can tie, count, and walk in place, and all with your eyes closed. Make up variations for yourself. Another added possibility is synchronizing your breathing in time with your walking, counting and tying.

The structural symmetry of the square knot is analogous to our anatomical symmetry. When your two legs are reasonably equal in length, strength, and agility, and the two lobes of your brain can easily commutate, you have a good start on great balance.

Knot tying can be intriguing and fun. Also, it is a great skill which impresses children. Knot tying is, of course, also good for children's brain development. Some jugglers have even combined knot tying with juggling. They create knots as if by magic, yet their knot-tying skills are nothing but the result of long practice. Tying any knot is very good for cross-lateral brain communication.

String Loop

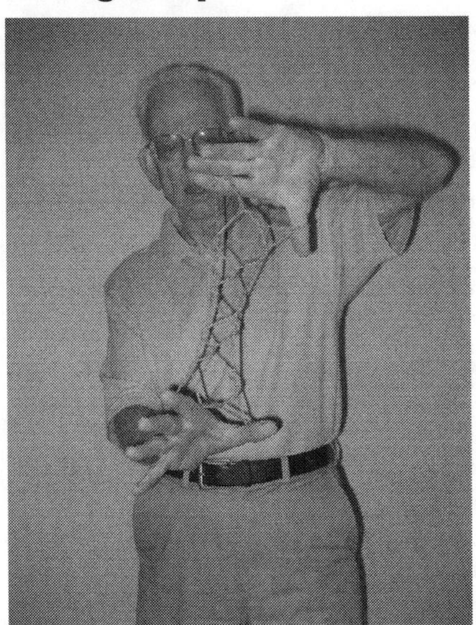

The Cat's Cradle is the most famous string game pattern. There are hundreds more, such as Cup and Saucer, Jacob's Ladder, Witches Broom, etc. String games are a great exercise for enhancing mental concentration, cross-lateral coordination, and brain-hand-eye interactions. This activity can be done any time, anywhere. The equipment is cheap, simple, and transportable. String manipulation is like knitting, although string tricks don't produce a permanent product. Also, string tricks encourage onlookers to share and to enter into the learning. Who knows, you might find a new friend as you climb the rungs of Jacob's ladder (pictured). Bookstores have books that will show you how to get started.

Play Piano

Play at the piano even though you can't play. At least pick out a tune. Use both hands as in Chop Sticks. Try Mary had a little Lamb, or make up a melody. Search out a chord that sounds good to you. Soon, Wow, Liberace . . . eat your heart out!

Pendulum

Tie a small ball or object to a string to make a pendulum. String is about 18 to 24 inches long. Hold the end of string and let your pendulum swing. Work out patterns, like a figure eight, or allow the pendulum to form a large U shape in front of you. In rhythm with the U pattern, allow your body to glide from side to side. Coordination between the upper and lower body is necessary for good balance. Another pattern is to let it swing from side to side, and then round in circles. Keep your eyes on the object on the end of the string. There is an infinite variety of patterns to invent.

Yo-yo

The yo-yo is not just for kids. It is a wonderful neurological challenge. Put the string on your middle finger. Start by merely dropping the yo-yo and getting it to come back up. The rhythm of the yo-yo is different from any other device. Hint: Just before the yo-yo reaches the bottom of the string your hand must rise to help the yo-yo rewind. It even helps to bend your knees at the right time to help the yo-yo to come back up. Find a young person to teach you more. He or she will be honored by your interest.

Spinning Top

You don't have to go around in circles with it, just get it going consistently. Practice and get better than a child in your life. Give him or her a top to spin and you two can practice together.

Faces

Make faces at yourself in the mirror. But especially, make faces with the children in your life. Let them copy you and vice versa. Smiles are the best way to make faces. I paraphrase, when your face smiles your whole self-smiles. Try it, that comedian in the mirror will make you laugh. What does making faces have to do with balance. A smiling, engaging face is the front for a more alert and beguiling mind. There is a connection between our attitude and that balanced life we all want.

Wink

Wink at people a lot, but only at those who will wink back. Use both eyes at different times. Make a wink part of your KAT practices. For example, walk and with every fourth footfall wink using a different eye. This is another form of concurrence and a way to gain control of your body. Disciplined control is part of balance. Your nervous system responds to these motor coordination challenges by becoming more responsible.

Tongue Twisters

Tongue Twisters are neurologically demanding. It is an achievement to learn a new one. The child in us loves them. Your tongue along with your mouth, larynx, lips, diaphragm, brain, and your willed intention, all work together to produce the complicated word sequencing.

The whole process from not knowing to knowing is a neurological integrative activity. Learn a tongue twister by itself, and then choreograph its rhythm with some motor activity. For example, as you walk you can say your tongue twister aloud and to the rhythm of the footfalls. Tongue twisters are akin to children's finger play; they challenge the brain to form new pathways. (See Appendix H for some tongue twister samples.)

Coin Off the Elbow

Bring your forearm up to a horizontal position at eye level with your elbow pointing forward. Your hand is near your ear, palm up. Place a coin or beanbag on your forearm very near the point of the elbow. Now suddenly lower your elbow. The coin will remain in the air for a short time, long enough to be caught by your hand on its downward stroke. The catching action is much like the crab, or catching flies. It's surprising how many people are successful in the first or second trial.

Advanced: Try two or more coins on the elbow and catch them all. Try this coin-catching trick with right hand and left hand. The trick goes so fast it looks like magic.

Coin Bombardier

Place a container on the floor. Taking a handful of pennies or pebbles, drop one at a time from standing height into the container. Do this from a stable, aiming position, and then make it harder by "bombing" as you walk by. Start with a large container and advance to a smaller one. Be sure the bomber uses both hands.

Some of these activities may seem silly. I guess they are on one level (I would rather think of them as plain fun), but anything you can practice to make your eyes, body, brain, and motivation that can award you protection from falls has got to be good. Never let the hint to silly get the way of serious goals.

The next tool will highlight the relationship between an activity that may appear silly on the surfaced, but it is fully serious. You will soon see what I mean.

52 Pick Up

Most people remember being tricked into playing 52 Pick Up when they were young. However, 52 Pick Up does have some redeeming qualities. The ability to bend down and touch the floor and then up again is a fantastic balance practice. Strength and flexibility are needed, and if you bend down repeatedly, it can be aerobic. Facetiously, I suggest becoming an obsessive lint picker-upper. Even better is making a useful balance exercise with the game of 52 Pick Up. To keep from slipping on the cards, drop the whole deck in a little-used corner.

The practice consists of picking up one card one at a time. An 80-year-old student tried the game at home and found all sorts of ways to make it more fun, as well as safe. His balance was precarious, so he began playing 52 Pick Up seated in a chair. He bent down, picked up one card at a time. He then advanced to standing with his back to the corner so if he pitched backward he was safe. He also put a solid chair in front of him if he needed assistance in getting up.

He found himself favoring his best hand for each pick up. So, he decided to pick up the first card with his right hand then the next with the left. After a while, he picked up one card with each hand simultaneously. Then he put down the cards all face up. He chose to pick one suit at a time, beginning with twos and ending with aces. He discovered many variations on 52 Pick Up. At first, he reported that he could pick up only a few cards in a session. But persistent practice paid off. He became noticeably stronger. He measured his progress by the number of cards he could pick up without a rest.

Sooner than he expected, he got rid of the chair and the corner and was picking up all 52 in one practice session. Obviously, his endurance and balance progressed together.

With this game, you always win, not because you are the only player, but because your middle, back and thighs will become stronger and more flexible. Strength and flexibility are crucial for good balance.

Here's a variation that perhaps only I would try. I place myself flat on my back with the deck of cards at my feet. To get a card I have to do a sit up, procuring one card at a time. I lie down again, stretch out my arms over my head and put the card down on the floor. Then another sit up and another card. What an exercise this is! But then my creativity leaps into action. There are many ways to get up to a sitting position. I shall leave you with the problem. Necessity will kick in and you will find all sorts of possibilities. I add, you surely don't have to follow my lead with this exercise. But you are strongly advised to follow your own still small voice that loudly says, it is time for you to *fully* recognize that your health is your only true wealth.

A ball in the hand, drop it,
then pick it up from the floor.
Do what you can,
then do a little bit more.

Drop it again
bend down all the way.
Just bending over
will help stop decay.

52 Pick Up?
It's a stupid old game.
But bending way down
will keep you from lame.
Don't you believe me?
Try it; you'll see.
To become more balanced
is a fitness key.

This is one lesson
of the Kinetic Arts many.

You can think up your ways
without spending a penny.

I trust you will do it
with gusto and zest.
And soon you'll be better
even better than your best.

You won't become perfect
but you can teach your grand tots
that you're really terrific
and that's a grand lots.

The Human Body as a Tool

It may be a stretch to think of the body as a tool. But it is easy enough to think of your hands as tools for manipulating the world, feet as tools for locomotion, and the heart as a pump.

Balance researchers tell us there are five exercises that are essential for good balance. They can be done in many different way several times a day. Each of the five is very different but all are designed to improve your balance. I have put these in a little poem for easy memorization.

Wag your head.
Wiggle your hips.
Reach down to the floor,
Then look up at your tips.
Now stand on one leg and shout zippity zip.

Note: The zippity zip is optional.

There is a way to play 52 Pick Up and perform all five of these in the process. It's always a challenge to work on ever better health enhancing habits.

Focus Sign

The words: "*This world will not work as well without me,*"
are printed on a regular-sized sheet of paper and placed at the end of the classroom. Each line is printed in smaller type as you progress down the page. Here is s simulation:

This world
will not work
as well
without
me.

Participants begin at the other end of the room taking a few steps, stopping and attempting to read as much as possible. As they move closer, they will see and understand more. This exercise is to challenge visual focusing and mental concentration. To make this more difficult, ask the participant to briefly focus on his or her thumbnail between each look. Visual accommodation between far and near is vital for balance.

Rubber Band Snap

With your palm facing down, place a rubber band on the end of your index or middle finger. Pull the other end of the rubber band back over the top of your hand and let it fly out in front of you. Aim so it lands where you can find it again. Rubber Band Snap can be played in your home or anywhere, like, your Doctor's waiting room. Now back to reality. The value is in the bending down and picking up, which is one of the five essential actions needed to enhance balance. (See the section, *The Human Body as a Tool,* for the five.) Also, there is some considerable skill in getting the band to travel a reasonable distance.

The metaphor between life and a rubber band is clear. Its elasticity is like our brain's ability to learn. The pull back is the effort it takes to learn. Letting go is the courage to "go for it. And where does a rubber band land? It lands at a distance in relation to the skill and effort you put forth. Moral: You can stretch yourself to learn, you can let go, and make mistakes. Mistakes are to learn from and, in the process, you too can go a long way toward your goals. All you need is to stretch yourself while being anchored to something solid. Then let go and leap into tomorrow. Leaping forward is not a flighty pursuit.

Head Clock Counting

In Head Clock Counting, your head becomes a clock face with your forehead the 12 and the 6 at the back of your head. Place a finger on the 12, and say "12" aloud. Then move your finger to 1 o'clock and so on, around your head. Now try it backwards. Perform the number sequence with your other hand. Make it harder by beginning at 1, and then with the same finger, touch the 7, then 2, then 8, and so on. Another pattern is to limit your counting-touching to even numbers, and then only to odd numbers. One man told me he alphabetized the numbers and touched them in that order. The aim is to keep the spaces between the numbers as even as possible.

> Note: in case you wish to try the numbers in alphabetic order, here they are:
> Eight Eleven Five Four Nine One Seven Six Ten Three Twelve Two

Use both hands. Put your right index finger on the 12 and your left index finger on the 6, and say aloud, "12" and then "6." Simultaneously move your right hand to 1 and your left to 7, and say "1" and "7." Keep going all the way around. Each time you say a number, increase the pressure a bit on that number, i.e. your head. This is a very personal exercise. It helps to close your eyes.

The value of Head Clock Counting is stimulation of the spatial brain centers in connection with the motor centers. Also, when you try this, you may well experience a meditative perspective.

Here is a *walking the clock* activity. Imagine a clock on the floor in front of you. It can be as large as you like. You are standing on the 12, facing the 6. Remember the number will appear upside down. Beginning with your left foot on number one, then right foot on two, and so on around the clock face. Transpose the numbers from upside down to right side up. You can walk the clock in many different combinations of number and stepping patterns. The child's game of hopscotch is something like Head Clock Counting.

If standing or walking is too difficult, sit and tap your feet on floor clock numbers. Be sure to alternate your feet on adjacent numbers. The two lobes of the brain are also working when you alternate your hands or feet in any action. We all have time to use our finger on our heads, or feet on the floor to touch imaginary clock numbers as a KAT tool to sharpen our spatial abilities.

Ice Cream Cone (ICC)

Remember, the three defenses against falls are your *ankles, hips, and step.* All three defenses help you retain your balance. The ICC and the next segment, the Wind Shield Wiper, concentrate on the ankle defense.

Stand with your feet comfortably apart. Stand in an erect position like a soldier at attention, with your arms at your sides. Performing the ICC in a doorway will provide security. Now rock slightly forward on your toes, then to the left, then on your heels, then to the right, and back to the front. Keep up this circular motion. The ICC is done without bending at the waist. Your head is the cone, and your feet the point of the cone. It's harder when you put your feet smack dab together.

It helps if you imagine your feet rooted into the floor. Keep your body calm but straight and tall. First, concentrate on the action of your ankles and feet. The Ice Cream Cone will strengthen your ankles and vividly let you know when your center of gravity is out of balance. Second, become aware of what the rest of your body is doing to retain its erect posture. Try it with shoes on and shoes off. You will feel the difference. Try the ICC with your eyes closed, but always be safe.

Just plain ankle circles are a great way to increase ankle muscles strength that you might have lost. Sit or lie and with one foot at a time, or both, make circles with your ankles. Rotate clockwise, then counterclockwise. Start with a few circles and gradually increase the number. Strong ankles will heighten your ankle's ability to do their balance job well.

Wind Shield Wiper (WSW)

Stand with both feet pointed straight ahead about inches apart. Lift your toes, and twist on your heels so your toes are pointed to the left. Then swivel again so your toes are pointed to the right. It's fun to make windshield wiper swishing sounds in time to the foot action. Like the Ice Cream Cone, the Windshield Wiper is good for strengthening the *Tibialis anterior* (the muscle is on the outside of the shinbone). This muscle needs to be strong so it will dutifully lift your toes over cracks in the sidewalks.

Finger Tracing

Put your left hand comfortably in front of you with your palm toward your right side. Your right index finger is touching the outside (the thumb side) of your left wrist. Begin tracing your left thumb up the outside, then down the other side, then up the index finger, and so on, up and down till you get to the outside of your little finger. Now repeat the tracing in the opposite direction. Keep the pressure and speed of your tracing the same throughout. You may wish to trace with a different finger for each sequence. Close your eyes and trace, but consciously sense which finger is being touched.

The coordination between breathing and hand tracing is a good example of concurrency, which tends to integrate the areas in the brain that control hands with the areas that control breathing. A very large brain area is dedicated to controlling the fingers and hands. The hands and fingers are also rich with sensory and motor nerves. When the hands touch each other, in any manner, the two lobes of the brain must coordinate their control duties. The coordination of any two body systems activates brain integration. This is a balance book that admits it is also a brain enhancement book.

One student said she liked to finger trace to music, eight beats per finger. Another student who has meditated for years said she finger traces to begin her meditation. Finger Tracing is a very calming experience which is introductory to the deeper meditative experience. She tells me she inhales while tracing toward the end of a finger then exhales on the way down. Meditation also focuses great attention on breathing. You can determine just how fast you wish to trace and breathe. Finger tracing brings your attention inward, promoting a calm state of mind. In this state, you can become more aware of who you really are. Equally important is that blood pressure can be lowered by calming yourself through any meditative exercise. No prescriptions or co-pay necessary. Better health is worth a try.

Finger Sensitivity (skin)

A coin is a good teaching device to stimulate finger sensitivity. At the same time, the brain areas that control the fingers are activated to sense differences in texture, pattern, size, etc. between heads or tails of a coin. Here are a few ways to heighten these abilities.

Start with a quarter. Look closely at both sides of each coin and visually identify the differences. Then close your eyes and feel what you know to be the heads side. Do the same on the tails side. Soon you will know the difference by feel. Many people are surprised by how fast they achieve success with just a few trials. Test yourself with different fingers on both hands. It helps to put your mind into your fingers, so to speak.

Next, concentrate on size alone. Place a quarter and a dime in your hand. Immediately you will feel the difference in their sizes and thickness. Now pair a penny, nickel, and dime with the quarter. Test out your skill. With practice, it is possible to sense the difference between heads and tails on all the coins, and at the same time, retrieve the coin you want from a pocket full of change.

While riding with a friend, I was fingering a coin. He asked what I was doing. I told him and he said, "Boy, you know how to get a cheap thrill." I thought, yes, it is a cheap thrill to know that this simple exercise is making my brain and my fingers more sensitive to the world around me.

In class, I make this coin exercise balance relevant by saying that an alert, and sensitive brain is a prerequisite for being aware of the potholes in life.

Here is another coin trick. Consult a magician or a book on magic and learn how to make a coin (or small ball) disappear. It is a coordinated move between the two hands and, thus, the two lobes of the brain. You don't have to be very good to fool small children. (the younger, the better) Then practice in front of a mirror. When you fool yourself, you are ready to show off. Of course, I'm being facetious, but mirrored practice can give you hints how to make your performance smoother.

The following 88 words will remind you of the many things that you can do with your fingers and hands. We are quite remarkable.

assail
assault
attack
bash
beat
belt
bend
caress
clench
clout
clutch
coddle
compact
compress
condense
constrict
contort
control
crunch
cuddle
cuff
defend
entwine
fidget
fondle
giggle
grab
grasp
grip
hit
intertwine
knock
lash
move
pack
pat
pick
pincer
pinch
press
pressure
pronate
punch
put
quiver
rotate
rub
salute
screw
seize
shake
shiver
shutter
signal
slip
smack
sock
squeeze
squirm
strike
stroke
supinate
swat
swipe
swirl
tamp
tap
thud
thump
thwack
touch
trap
tremble
turn
twist
vibrate
waffle
waggle
wallop
wave
whack
wiggle
wipe
wobble
worm
wring
writhe
write

Wrist and Body Twisting

The purpose here is to encourage the shoulders into a full range of motion. Grasp your right wrist with your left hand. Then slowly twist both hands and arms in opposite directions. When you reach your limit, come back the other way. It takes a little strategy to see how far you can really go.

Moshe Feldenkrais, an Israeli physicist studied human body mechanics and kinesiology. He invented a therapeutic approach that bears his name. One of his many exercises is a twisting exercise, concentrating on head, shoulders and hips. Stand tall. Slowly turn your head to the right while simultaneously turning your shoulders to the left. Then reverse the directions of the head and the shoulders till you can repeatedly perform this coordinated move smoothly and effortlessly.

Now add the hips. The hips turn in the same direction as the head while the shoulders turn in the opposite direction.

Brain integration greatly expands when the body is challenged to learn new and evermore complex motor patterns. If at first you do not succeed, try try again. The little engine that *could* will be proud of you.

Triangle and Square

Draw a square about two inches on a side. To the right of the square, draw a triangle, with the point on the top and as tall as the square. Place your left index finger on the upper-right corner of the square and your right index finger on the top point of the triangle. Now, in unison, move your left finger straight down the side of the square and your right finger down the right slope of the triangle. Trace around the square and the triangle 12 times. Count the lines as you go. Because the square has four sides and the triangle has three it will take 12 moves to allow your fingers to end up at the same time at their beginning points. Repeat this till you can trace the square and triangle in the air. Ask your friends to try it. They will be amazed that you can do this without looking at the paper. The right and left brain lobes are working magnificently together to perform this spatially oriented feat.

Double Doodles (DD)

Double Doodles is an exercise in body-brain symmetry. Practically, DD helps you become more ambidextrous. Stand at a chalkboard with chalk or markers in both hands. Draw with both hands at the same time, tracing the same pattern with your right hand and your left. You will find that your lesser-used hand follows the other very well, proving that you are more ambidextrous than you thought.

Cursive letters, numbers and words may be dual-scribed. It is said that DD will help make your writing more legible. Make your drawings with extreme movements of both hands and body. Bigger is better. Without a blackboard, use a large sheet of paper on a table or drawing in the air is an alternative.

Normally a person will allow the best hand to take the lead. KAT suggests focusing, from time to time, on the least preferred hand, demand that it take the lead. This is an excellent cross-lateral exercise where concentration is consciously shifted from the dominant brain lobe to the other.

You can draw pictures. Try a Christmas tree beginning at the top, using both hands at the same time. Then try a frontal view of a face. Writing your name in big cursive letters requires physical movement from left to right. The finished product is both names superimposed on each other. To avoid this, lower one hand a bit and raise the other. There is much room for experimentation with Double Doodles.

Chopsticks

Using sticks for eating seems a little strange to many Americans. But when the occasion arises, try them. Ask the waiter for a little help. The mere act of willingly trying something very different is good for the body and brain as well as being a good sport.

Hoop

A large embroidery hoop or hula-hoop is an intriguing tool. Place your arm inside the hoop. Get it moving in a circle around your arm with the help of your free hand. To keep it going, move your arm up and down. See how long you can keep it in motion.

A regular hula-hoop is especially great for a special game you can play by yourself. Point the hoop ahead of you and toss it out a short distance. But, just before you let go, put reverse spin on it. The friction of the reverse spin will make the hoop come back to you. The child in us all loves tricks that look like magic. When children ask why does it do that, you can explain *friction.*

Origami

Paper cutting and folding is an excellent practice for developing manual dexterity. Also, inherent in Origami is a lot of problem solving. It is an especially good workout for the spatial areas of your brain. And the product you create is arty and fun.

Exercises for Vertigo

Vertigo is a serious medical condition, requiring professional neurological attention. The difficulty is that as we get older our inner ear apparatus gives out and we don't move our head in space like we did when we were young. Even the inner ear needs to be used to keep fit. Persons with vertigo are advised to use caution when exercising.

When the head is quickly tilted up, down, or sideways, the inner ear reacts. Sometimes, the reaction includes dizziness, nausea, or worse. Balance is precarious when an attack comes on suddenly.

The inner ear, in all of us, is healthier when used. If you have vertigo, here is a safe and stable position to exercise up to your limits. Sit down in a chair or stand with your back in a corner with your feet widely spaced. Now even if you become dizzy or fall backwards, you will not go far. Always exercise with some forethought for safety.

There are some preventative exercises to keep those semi-circular canals in the inner ear as healthy as possible. Keep your head and neck moving. This means to look up and down, from side to side, move your head in diagonals as in an X. Swimming is helpful, because the water allows you to move your head in various orientations. Bending to the floor to pick something up is good exercise for the inner ear. Watching a tennis game from the side demands that you quickly turn your head from side to side to follow the play. Watching on TV does not count.

The V warm-up exercise, where you move a ball slowly while focusing intently on it, is a good inner-ear exercise. In fact, tossing a ball up in the air requires you to keenly follow it with your eyes and head to predict just where to put your hand to catch it. Your whole body takes part in the catching process, not just your hand. Shifting your weight is part of catching, and your inner ear is most helpful in allowing this process to be accomplished.

Let me emphasize that if you have inner ear problems see a professional. Many of these difficulties can be ameliorated.

Groups

A group is considered a tool in itself. Working with others is a joy when there is shared purpose. Sociality is an intimate human trait. Groups provide an incentive to 'get on with it'. Below are several balance-oriented activities that can be done in pairs or a group.

Ask a group to alphabetize themselves in a circle by the first letter in their first name. Let the group solve the organizational problems of just where in the circle to place the As Bs etc, and whether to order the letters clockwise or otherwise. The first trial always demonstrates confusion. Ask them to think of ways to do it faster and easier. Then change the request and alphabetize according to the first letter in their last name. Groups always become more process efficient with practice. Use this activity as an analogy in how the nervous system becomes more organized with practice. Other ordering criteria might be height, or birthdays or anything the group can think of. This is a great group game at family parties.

Notice that each person must place him or herself with regard to everyone else. They must walk carefully to avoid others, and they must understand the over all-purpose of the ordering. Problem solving is part of balance.

Here's another group exercise called a Knot Group. Ask everyone in the circle to walk toward the middle till there is a tight knot of people. Now they are asked to move, this way and that, avoiding others, but staying within the same small space. They might say hello to people they meet. The leader could even suggest they shake hands with whomever they meet. You will find that shy persons insist on staying the outside of the knot. They will warm up . . . eventually.

Have them form a circle again. Now, each person, at the same time, moves to the other side of the circle. I call this the Walk Through. This is a problem-solving activity that demands cooperation, timing, and consideration of others. Do this more than once. They will soon create easier and faster ways to perform the position exchange.

From the circle, ask the group to do the wave, like they do at sporting events. Help them start by designating the beginning person. Each person begins his or her wave action with bended knee, slight for those with knee pain. Straighten knees, come up on toes and raise both hands when the time comes. Here again, each person must be alert to the group goals and do his or her part at the right time. Attention is part of balance.

How about a square or line dance? Swing your partners is an easy one. A modified Rockette chorus line is very social. Adjacent persons in a circle place their arms around their neighbors. Designate a well-rhythmed person in the circle to be the leader. They do the counting for the steps. High kicks are not needed. Suggest each person kick up or do toe touches according to his/her ability. The goal is to stay in unison with the group.

A circle is a good structure to perform some familiar tongue twisters or songs, choral style. A double circle instantly created partners who can converse as they walk around in the circle. Couples can waltz, shake hands in creative ways, or tell jokes. The longer a group is together, the more family-like they become. Encouragement to learn ever more is a family responsibility.

Clickers

Remember those thumb-activated, press-and-release clicking devices we had when we were kids? They were no more than an inch or so in length, with a piece of spring steel as the only moving part. When a clicker is pressed down it clicks and when released it clicks again. It is a beautiful tool whose sharp sound is a direct response to finger activation. Even people who are hard of hearing can respond to its sharp beat.

A clicker is like finger snapping. Use it whenever a self-initiated rhythm is desired. You can coordinate the clicking with aloud counting, or the cadence of words, or each footfall. Then try two clicks for each footfall. Keep the rhythm even. Keep time to music with your clicker. Recite a poem with the clicker responding to the poem's meter. With children or even with some adult groups, place the clicker in your pocket and, as a joke, click it at an opportune moment. Make people wonder where the sound is coming from.

Click with one hand and with the other slap to the hip. A clicker in each hand makes it more neurologically complicated. Click with left hand on right footfall, and a right hand click on left footfall. Two hands and two feet have to work together to follow the demands of cross-lateral action. Sense the beat of music and click and move with some personality. When you are alone, what do you care what it looks like. If you don't have a clicker, snap your fingers. The goal, of course, is to make neurological integration a fun and learning sport.

Respiration

For centuries, practitioners of Yoga, Tai Chi and meditation have espoused the value of proper breathing. Respiration is automatic, however, it may also be consciously controlled. In this regard, your breathing cycles may be coordinated with walking. Try inhaling on four steps, then exhaling on four steps. Modify the rhythm according to your need. Then add a wink on a designated footfall. And don't forget language. Poetry is rhythmic; its meter may be incorporated into the overall walking-breathing pattern. Turning your head from side to side, clenching your hands, and/or snapping your fingers are more possibilities. Again, the more concurrent action the better. Doing more than one thing at a time enhances brain functioning and body coordination. Each time a new neurological pattern is learned the brain builds new connections and pathways. A good brain will keep you safe.

Kinetic Arts equipment often seems rinky-dink,
But all its tools encourage integrative think.

Balance Tests (A Partial List)

Below are five simple tests with which you can keep track of your balance progress. You are encouraged to use them for practice toward better balance. The goal is to determine your present ability level, and then practice to make your scores better and better. Even if your ability does not increase, as you get older, at least you are holding your own in the face of advancing age. But oft times, ability increases. The outcome of enhanced balance ability is more strength, agility, balance, and most of all a feeling of well being from becoming more neurologically fit. Fewer falls is the bottom line.

<u>Get Up and Go</u>

- *Preparations:* A chair is placed eight feet from a cone or a mark on floor. This is a timed test. See below.
- *Directions*: Sit in the chair, get up, walk around the mark, and sit back down.
- *Measurement*: Begin timing when your backside leaves the chair and stop timing when you sit down again. Someone else may time you with the second hand. Or a metronome, set on one second per beat, will give you a good idea of time. Mere counting is better than nothing but is a rough measure at best.
- *Value*: How long it takes to do this exercise will give you an idea of how precarious your balance is. The longer this activity takes, the more precarious your balance is. As you increase your speed in the test, your balance becomes more secure. This is a dynamic test of control, strength and balance. It is also a test of your ability to come up with a good strategy to learn to do things better.

Hint: It takes less time to get out of the chair when you begin by sitting on the edge of the chair. Before the timer says, "Go," bend forward like a sprinter. Place your feet so you can get right off the mark. Decide if you are going to the left or right around the mark.

<u>Fifty Steps</u>

- *Preparation*: Place a piece of tape on the floor at least 10 feet from a wall or obstruction.
- Directions: Stand on the taped spot, close your eyes and take 50 steps, standing in place and counting aloud on each footfall. You have two goals. The first is to try to remain at your starting spot as you walk in place. If you have met the second goal, you will still be facing the same wall.
- *Measurements*: Two measurements may be taken: the distance in inches you move from the beginning spot and your change in direction from the beginning orientation.
- *Value*. The very fact you can close your eyes and step in place is of great value to enhancing the somatosensory system. After practice, you will be able to control yourself more and stay in the same place without turning or moving from the spot. If your are afraid to try this, touch a wall with one hand as you step or, better yet, stand in a doorway and touch the door jambs on both sides. If for any reason you are unsteady during the test, open your eyes. Also, at first it is a good idea to have someone else present.

Standing on Foam Rubber
- *Preparation*: Stand on a solid floor, with your arms folded across your chest.
- *Directions*: Phase One - 1. Stand still on both feet with your eyes open for 30 seconds. 2. Stand with your eyes closed for 30 seconds.
  Phase Two – 1. Stand on a soft foam-rubber surface with your eyes open for 30 seconds. 2. Stand with your eyes closed for 30 seconds.
- *Measurements*: The length of time the directions can be followed.
- *Value*: When your eyes are closed, you must rely on your somatosensory system to tell you what to do to keep your balance. The somatosensory system needs exercise to keep active and able.

Functional Reach
- *Preparation*: A yardstick is taped horizontally on a wall about chest high. A vertical line is drawn upward from the low numbered end of the yardstick.
- *Directions*: Stand erect, parallel to the wall, with arms outstretched. Position yourself so that your fingertips are right at the vertical line and the yardstick is in sight. Without moving your feet, bend forward at your waist as far as possible without losing balance.
- *Measurements*: The number of inches covered by the forward bend without falling forward.
- *Value*: The second defense against falls is hip flexibility. The more flexible your hips are, the better you can maintain your center of gravity in case of an emergency.

Chair Ups
- *Preparation*: Sit on the edge of a hard chair. Fold your arms across your chest with both feet solidly on the floor. (This position may be altered, depending on your conditions). Directions: Quickly rise from the chair to a full standing position, and then sit again.
- *Measurements*: Count the number of times you can get up and (sit down), in 30 seconds.
- *Value*: The quadriceps, the muscles in the front of your thighs, are strengthened, your aerobic capacity is increased, your balance is challenged each time you stand and sit, and your determination is enhanced by competing with yourself to increase the number of chair ups in 30 seconds. Perform more than once a day.

I began this book with a quote from Buckminster Fuller, mathematician, poet, philosopher, engineer, and creative futurist. In his book, *I Seem to be a Verb,* where by a verb stands for action, and action is the energy of life. You become a verb when you live yourself as an action verb in your own life's script.

The environment to each must be
every thing that isn't me.
The universe in turn must be
everything that isn't me . . . plus me.
Fuller

Your *life-long health* is important, your *balance* is crucial,
and indeed, your *very being* is of unique value.

Epilogue

Balance is Like an Olympic Sport

Kinetic Arts balance is a way of thinking
about this fabulous journey we call life.
Life is an art, of which we are a part.
We are more than flecks of paint on a Universal canvas.
We are more than a chunk of alabaster,
and much more than the sculpture.
We are more than a click of a camera,
and are more than a mere image.
We are more, much more than we think
or can think, or even know.

We can be more than we have ever been.
We can be more than we are right now.
We can be more than anyone knows.
We can be more than more . . .
with minds that can soar.

Our gift is to control
much of what we become.
Our decisions, or behaviors,
or goals, our hopes and fears
all play through us.
At any age, we are allowed to travel
the path we choose as life.

Our persistence is our paint.
Our patience is our canvas.
Our practice is our brush, along with our fingers,
our hands, our heart and our mind.
We are a masterpiece ready to burst forth.

There is absolutely no end to the better in us.

Acknowledgements

All kinds of people have influenced my life, and all have become a direct and indirect part of it. They are listed alphabetically by first name.

Alan Anderson, our Carthage College breakfast club leader, who remains a leader.
Alan Watts, a philosopher who loved to crack your head open with ponderous thoughts.
Alice Jones, my high school English teacher. She treated me like I had a brain.
Alice Kibby, a biologist and curmudgeon whose funny voice stated serious thoughts.
Bill Rapp, my father, who sent me to college against all odds of graduation.
Bob Carius, a high school colleague whom I always admired.
Britt Poulson, educator, movie buff, editor-advisor, and more than friend.
Buckminster Fuller, mathematician, philosopher, engineer, and motivator of thought.
Bud Rasmussen, educator, administrator, and stalwart practitioner of personal sovereignty.
Coco Readdick, long time friend, astute editor, and valued connection to the CD world.
David Felder, philosopher, writer, and facilitator of the written word.
Elmer Craeger, friend, inventor, original thinker, and much more.
George Barnard, Forensic Psychiatrist, and daring inventor of Motoric Therapy,
Harold Sutton, art educator, extraordinary thinker, and motivator.
Herb Gould, my high school coach, who allowed me to play quarterback on our first high school football team. Coaching rendered him a great school superintendent.
Irv Jahns, adult educator, terrific friend, ideational advisor and fantastic sounding board.
Jack Stumpf, my bowman who trusted me to steer the canoe.
Jerry Maitland, a Neurologist, and valued advisor on balance issues.
Jesse Wilson, carpenter, an impressive lion of a man.
Jessie Jones, balance researcher-writer, who share with me valuable balance ideas.
Joyce Williams, long time colleague, courageous friend, precise editor and more.
Juanita Jones, delightfully jolly World Lit teacher who enthusiastically modeled the wonders of literary analysis.
Julian Greenly, science educator, and provocateur of the deepest of thoughts.
Kathy Neu, who trusted my work and allowed me in to instruct my first full class.
Lynn Panton, an energetic researcher physiologist and teacher with a fabulous future.
Marvin Rosenblatt, a child psychologist who encouraged a one-time, self-doubter.
Michael Rogers, a balance researcher who is very clever and inventive.
Nancy Spears, friend and hospital volunteer coordinator and appreciator of us older ones.
Nora Jane Hendrickson, stalwart lover and protector of the Democratic process.
Ralph Hurst, artist, sculptor, and conveyer of profound thoughts.
Randy Vickers, creatively offers Solutions Skills to all of us learners.
Ruth Dales, my major professor, an academic undercover agent of the very best kind.
Suzy Fay, my 'look me in the eye' editor. We agreed 99.44/100 percent of the time.
Those special, still-remembered high school dance dates who jitterbugged up a storm.
Tom Hart, noteworthy friend, who gave his valuable time in the formatting process.
Tonya Toole, ardent motor-control learning researcher who willingly answered my questions.
Walter Bortz, writer, inspirational speaker, 50-Plus-fitness ambassador, *extraordinary*.
Wayne Strunk, my high school critic, who made me think that I might end up something.
To all my balance class members who want what they once had.

I honor all those negative people, ideas, situation and thoughts that I chose *not* to follow. I respectfully dedicate this book to all who wish to prolong their neurological health into their later years. Specifically, to the elderly, the injured and disease and not to omit those couch potatoes, who need and desire the riches of independence.

I could never leave out Westminster Oaks Retirement Community where I taught my first two classes, the Tallahassee Senior Citizens Center which allowed me to teach balance in their beautiful space, and to Len Harvey, director of the Tallahassee Premier Health and Fitness Center who understood the need for a balance class. Premier was one of the first gyms in the nation to create a dedicated balance class.

Biography for Don Rapp, Ph.D.

Learned to juggle in 1940 at 12 years of age

Extensive High School and College Sport participation

Carthage College BS in Physical Education

Physical Therapy Technician, US Army

Florida State University Elementary School certification

Florida State University MS, Early Childhood Education

First male public school kindergarten teacher in the State of Florida

Paris American High School dormitory counselor, Paris, France

Florida State University, Ph.D., Child Development

Taught at University of Illinois, University of Georgia, and Florida State University, Child Development, Gerontology, and Creativity for 34 years.

Year long Behavioral Science Psychiatric fellowship at Shands Medical Center, Gainesville, Florida

Two guest appearances on the Mr. Roger Neighborhood show. One performing a juggling 'concert' and the other on the value of Bean Bags for young children.

American College of Sports Medicine member and certification as an exercise leader and personal trainer.

Become Your Own Balance Coach, (A Kinetic Arts Balance manual), 2000

Author: On Balance Mastery of Physical Balance for Life

Employed by the Tallahassee Regional Medical Center Premier Health Center to teach a Kinetic Balance class, 2000 – date.

Kinetic Arts Instructor (Juggling) summer counselor for the Chautauqua Boys and Girls Club for second grade through teen-age 1998 – date.

Appointed to the Florida Governor's Council on Physical Fitness.

Continues to speak on balance enhancement and the tools of creative thought.

Don Rapp may be reached at the web Rappdp@aol.com

Habit Busters

These 83 Habit Busters are powerful behaviors that can break ineffective habits. Habit Busters make you think. They even make your body think. They bring you to full consciousness and render you ready to learn ever better habits. Habit Busters always have a physical and attitudinal component. They tell you that you are too habitual, too customary, too rigid in your ways of thinking and doing. They are like bumps in the night. To be creatively balance you must to be ready to move to the next pattern of thought. After you have read the following and tried a few, make up others that will help you become the person you want to become. A few suggested Habit Busters.

With your lesser hand brush teeth, open doors, drink coffee, scissors, etc. / Learn to juggle. /Play a musical instrument./ Walk as a dance, think rhythm./ Dance to music in your living room in your underwear. . . no holes please. / Learn child finger plays. / Give a $ to a rich friend. / Pollute creatively, i.e., be nice to everyone/ Experiment with your budget, spend less. / Lock yourself out of your house then get in. (plan ahead). / Junk the junk food. / Drink water instead of soft drinks. / Buy a self-help book and read it for a change. (Note the double meaning.) / Have a tantrum about your too frequent tantrums. / Eat with chopsticks, learn to love'em. / Wake up your teenagers with breakfast in bed; now they will know what to love your for. / Praise a speaker before s/he begins. / Draw something even if you think you cannot. / Withdraw only one $ from your checking account and buy something which gives you pleasure. / Send a check for $20 to a friend, and then negotiate how they must earn it. / Fix something you said you couldn't (or wouldn't). / Placate your guilt by apologizing, or paying retribution. / Praise yourself when you do right, (and if you don't know what is right, don't call me). / Brag that you are a good person, then behave better than your bragging. / Watch TV for only the good stuff (you define the good). / Be early to an appointment. / Love your boss, even when s/he's cross (hate can be your albatross). / Learn something from children. / Wash your hands separately, one at a time. / Plan with everyone's success in mind. / Insist on only win-win situations. / Go without your glasses for a while. / Breath only clean fresh air (stop smoking). / Talk only in Rhyme. / At home for one full day wear only a towel, (one that goes with your eyes). / Laugh and cry at the same time. / Look at your naked self in a full-length mirror right after a shower . . . try not to laugh. / Say out loud you LOVE your work. Remember that repetition is good. / Loudly say hello to a tree, the morning sun & your brain's unused capacity. / Nod your head to any positive self-affirmation. / Say thank you to a compliment. / Put your pajamas on inside out and go to bed. You won't sleep inside out. / For just one night, sleep with your head at the foot of the bed. / Say the alphabet backwards. / Stand on a chair and recite a poem. / For a day don't wear your watch. You'll be surprise how many nice ways you can ask for the time. / Sit in a different seat than usual. / If you usually eat with TV on, turn it off. / Have each family member take turns waiting on the family table, leave tip. / Change radio station you usually listen to. / Wear a hat to church, Male and Female. / Write a letter instead of phoning. / Start grocery shopping in produce rather than the reverse. / Turn on classical tapes in the presence of your country-loving friend. / Be ready first on Sunday morning. / Part your hair on the opposite side. / Forget your umbrella, just get wet. Walk around your house blindfolded. / Read the table of contents of five books, interrelating what you think you know from the five books. / Spoon honey up with a fork. / Brush your hair with your toothbrush. Point to your elbow and say knee. / Wave with your foot. / Try writing with your less dominate hand. / Clean the house clockwise and then counter clockwise. / Put lemon on your salad instead of dressing. / Park farther from the store and walk. / Really do what is on your 'to do' list. / Drive the speed limit for once. / Read the last chapter in a book first. / Wear two different colored socks. / Eat breakfast for dinner, dinner for breakfast. / Wear sunglasses inside and to bed. / Wear your belt backwards. / Sleep during the day and stay up all night. / Invite an enemy over for tea. / Drive to a well-known destination in a new way. / Change perfume. / Put on make up in the dark. / Eat with your fingers. / Sit in you dinner chair with back to front. / Read a book all the way through. / Meditate instead of procrastinate. /

Stages of Learning

Ray Gottlieb is a Behavioral Optometrist in Rochester, NY. He is creative in his teaching and works with all levels from the athlete to the mentally handicapped. He suggests that knowing his stages of learning accelerates your learning process. These five questions are on a graded scale. Ask yourself:

Can I do it?
Can I do it well?
Can I do it well for a long time?
Can I do it well for a long time in the face of distractions?
Can I do it creatively?

Learning takes practice. Practice requires a commitment to rehearsal time, which can often be done within your daily routine. A good attitude about yourself, in relation to practice is essential. If you don't like the word practice, call it rehearsal, or maybe:

Body-mind exercises
Central nervous system augmentation
Learning program
Performance drills
Preparation for perfection
Self-enhancement activities
Self-teaching
Training
Trial runs
Or make up your own. But make it positive.

Comment: When the light at the end of the tunnel is in sight, one has renewed motivation to get on with the task. Each of the five questions above is a tunnel in itself. There is light at the end of each. And that is the way these questions work. When you know just where you are on this five-point scale, you can work toward the next step. Intermediate goals are good. Life is but one step at a time.

When you don't show up for practice, there is no show.

Kinetic Arts Training Principles

Learning is better accomplished when one's philosophical readiness is up to the challenge. Embedded in Kinetic Arts Training are repeated considerations of positive philosophies. Some of these principles are KAT specific while others are for general health.

Learning is not all in your head.
Discouragement is never an option.
Patience and persistence work together.
Flexibility - learn to learn from your mistakes.
Repetition, adjustment, and flexibility are good.
People are important, choose your teachers wisely.
Goal setting is the beginning of the future you want.
Fun is a basic nutrient for mental and physical health.
Adjustment means it is ok to change (change is normal).
Positive affirmations remind you often of what you want.
Admit the problem, fix it, and reward your best behavior.
Visualization is seeing what you want before you have it.
Complicated skills are best learned when you start simple.
General health enhancement is a vital part of motor fitness.
Personal responsibility is the capacity to be fully trustworthy.
Use the past to plan your future, but best, live in the present.
Kinetic Arts Axiom - Do what you can, then a little bit more.
Self-control may be practiced by varying the speeds of motor action.
Concurrency means to practice doing more than one thing at a time.
Repetitious practice etches the practiced skill into new brain patterns.
Praise yourself only when you've done something better than yesterday.
Individuation-Integration: Both Micro and Marco events are important.
Attention switching means to practice alternating sensory focus quickly.
Our brain is capable of forming new pathways until the moment of death.
Every part of the body contributes to or detracts from successful learning.
The Wonder factor gives birth to the zest of awe, amazement, and surprise.
Regression is good when the past is used to learn quickly like a creative child.
Get serious about personal betterment then it becomes a ski slope to the goal.

These 28 principles are some philosophic bits talked about in Kinetic Arts Training. Even if you are not training in any form, these principles are an interesting lot to contemplate.

A comment on the stepwise process of learning. Learning begins with intention, and if strong enough becomes a wish, then a want, then a desire and finally a will. If your powers are willful enough, action ensues and eventually interactions. The process promotes the possibility of learning, and thus the etching of new neural pathways.

Just a thought: The statement, discouragement is never an option, is not to be confused with the military like statement that says defeat is never an option. You can make a realistic decision to retreat. But discouragement can never be part of the decision equation.

Growing Young Traits

Growing Young, a book by Ashley Montagu, gives 26 child traits that too many of us toss out as we grow up. He suggests we go back and get them for our health, our creativity, and for our very life.

1. THE NEED FOR LOVE - The more your give the more you get.

2. FRIENDSHIP - If you like yourself, you have one friend for sure.

3. SENSITIVITY - The ability to deeply and finely perceive, feel, and be competent in human relationships. Practice makes perfect.

4. THE NEED TO THINK SOUNDLY - The brain is nourished by the symphony of life. Self-orchestration consists of prudent choices and thoughtful decisions.

5. THE NEED TO KNOW - Involvement, acquisition, and discrimination, all generate knowing. Knowing endows sensation with meaning.

6. THE NEED TO LEARN – Become aware of what you know and what your don't know. The gulf between the two is always vast. Learning makes it jumpable.

7. THE NEED TO WORK - Work is the connection between intention and the end product. Work adds a conscious dimension to our survival biology. Work is decisioned direction.

8. THE NEED TO ORGANIZE - The human mind collects, arranges, and classifies its perceived universe. All minds are unique organizers.

9. CURIOSITY - Curiosity never stays on the path. The curious mind is a rich brain forest of possibilities. Healthy curiosity is a mind always growing in happenings. Be curious about your own brain -- both left and right. Our boss mind is infinitely more than our slave brain. The mind is the boss of the mind. The mind has a mind of its own.

10. THE SENSE OF WONDER - Wonder is an exaltation of interest and excitement, plus the expectation of 'more to come'. Wonder's diet is the unknown, i.e. every luscious bite of it.

11. PLAYFULNESS - Play always surprises and transcends mere repetition. Play need not be competitive, i.e., losing or winning. Rather, it is the drafting of time into joy and radiating creativity, which has long been patented as life.

12. IMAGINATION - "As if" is imagination's body, play is imagination's fingers, and mind is imagination's tool to conjure, pretend, dream, and create.

13. CREATIVITY - Creativity is best served as a sandwich. Top slice = imagination, bottom slice = thought. And in the middle is a laminated lean steak of passion and discipline. Our free will can choose a diet of nourishing ideas.

14. OPEMMINDEDNESS - A closed door disallows insight. An open mind has many doors, and they all have well-greased hinges. The only lock is on the inside. An open mind throws a party for ideas of promise.

15. FLEXIBILITY - Human adaptability is tri-segmented. 1. For others with the words empathy and consideration. 2. For ones own abilities of insight and inventions. 3. For the inanimate which is represented in atoms and their arrangements, which incredible become our cells as well as our tools and brains. (However, I feel duty bound to suggest that the universe, by quantity, is weighted more to the inanimate than the animate).

16. EXPERIMENTAL-MINDEDNESS – A good science, trial and error, and a billion probes, each with a million fingers. Busy, busy, don't stop it or crop it.

17. EXPLORATIVENESS - Examine every closed door, every hidden core, and the means to some day soar. Fathom deeply, and dig everywhere. The process is in the practice, and the product is in the new paradigm that erases present limits.

18. RESILIENCY - Children have more bounce per ounce than adults. And our childhood frame is always present. Bounce before you hit bottom. Revisit the resiliency of your childhood. There are many ways to bounce.

19. THE SENSE OF HUMOR - To laugh *at* others is sick. To laugh *with* others is health for both. However, to laugh at oneself is to open your future too much more than a mere bit of wit.

20. JOYFULNESS - Competition is fully enjoyed only by the winner. Co-operation is "win-win". Win-win makes the game a party in which the teams and the audience join to share in the collective score.

21. LAUGHTER AND TEARS - Laughter as well as tears release tensions from the body, while the same laughter and tears focus the attention of the mind. Laughter is an outburst of encapsulated zest, while tears search for meaning. You are invited to belly up to laughter's bar while enjoying your tears, which are generated by the cinema of your life.

22. OPTIMISM - Positive trending happens when you optimize your perception in three ways: 1. Knowing what really is. 2. Visualizing your goals. 3. Know want you want and what is healthy. The connection is textured with hope, generalized as planning and action toward your goal. Optimism is perseverance in search of its own reward.

23 HONESTY AND TRUST - Honesty sees reality on one side and fantasy sees it on the other. Both sides are healthy, as long as you honestly know the difference between reality and fantasy.

24. COMPASSIONATE INTELLIGENCE - Compassion and intelligence are both companions of growth . . . which gently reads aloud to itself. And as its reading progresses, a logical passion arises to call itself Integrity.

25. DANCE - Rhythm is basic . . . a time to live, a time to die. I'll do the math, if you'll bake the pie. Dancing alone is ok. Dancing with another is even greater. But when the nation dances, emotional repressions become a national expression of glorious health.

26. SONG - We are all natural singers and hummers. Sing your song loud and clear; steer clear of stage-fright fear. Sing as the drum major, the band director, and the band. When we sing we all strut in our own parade.

Category definitions by Don Rapp. Traits from Montagu, A., *Growing Young*. McGraw-Hill, Co., New York, 1981.

Rapp's Rap and Suggested Choreography

Rapp's Rap is the refrain from a Rap written for teenagers. It has proven to be ageless in its appeal.

This is my day I have arrived.
I'm a-kickin, I'm a-smilin, I'm alive I'm alive.
My future is assured, cause I can do it.
My future is me, ooh let me get to it.

I'm a-growin like mad , I'm a-learnin new things,
that make my brain like real steel springs.
I'm becomin I'm begoin I'm right for the job.
When I do my life right . . . shish-kebab.

Below are the words and their corresponding body motions found to be appropriate for the meaning of the words. The coordination between the motor, the linguistic, the word meaning and the confidence for showmanship is an example of the Kinetic Arts goal of brain-body integration.

This is my day,
With both hands and fingers pointed toward your chest.

I have arrived.
Step forward with arms up and out in pride of self.

I'm a-kickin, I'm a-smilin, I'm alive, I'm alive.
Kick, then point to your mouth, then arms up over head and out.

My future is assured,
Arms outstretch pointing in the distance to your future.

Cause I can do it.
Point to chest and touch it on cause, and do it. Also, continue with the same touch rhythm on the underlined words on the next line.

My future is me,
Point to your chest.

ooh,
While fingers are on your chest, bring elbows in vigorously to sides on the ooh.

let me get to it.
Keep elbows tight to the side.

I'm a-growin like mad,
Hands down in front of hip, with palms up, bring arms up toward sides of head.

I'm a learning' new things, that make my brain
Tap one index finger on your temple four beats on underlined words

like real steel springs.
Make a spiral, like a spring, with right finger pointing up by your temple.

I'm becomin',
Step short step to right.

I'm begoin',
Step short step to left.

I'm right for the job.
Ok sign with thumb and index finger forming a circle.

When I do my life right
One arm with elbow bent, upper arm touching chest, and hand just below the chin. The middle three fingers are curled in the palm of hand, while little finger and thumb stretched out. The hand begins close to the chest. Pulse outward on when and second pulse out on life. Then short pause . . .

. . . **shish-ka-bob!**
On shish, hand remains in the same position by chin, but elbow goes up to the horizontal while the hand remains by the chin. Then on ka-bob, elbow pivots down.

Now take your bow.

I guarantee all will have a good time performing Rapp's Rap. Courage to try it with a group comes with knowing you learn a lot by teaching others.

Kinetic Arts for the Tongue

(Make up body motion with the rhythms.)

Pimlico Pamlico pumpkins and peas.
Pepper them properly or you will sneeze.
Pop in a pipkin and bake until one.
Pimlico Pamlico then they'll be done.

If you saw a pink pug puppy playing with a pig,
or a great gray goose a golfing with a goat.
Would you think it half as funny as a big brown bunny,
blowing bubbles with a Bishop in a boat?

Chop chop, chopity chop.
Chop off the bottom and chop off the top.
What there is left we'll pop in the pot.
Chop chop chopity chop.

Beatty Batter bought some butter.
Put the butter in the batter made the batter bitter.
So, Beatty Batter bought some better butter
Than the bitter butter
put the better butter in the batter
made the batter better.

I'm an Irish Setter go-getter pace-setter.
My four legs are better much better than two.
I'm a setter who was never never a setter.
I'm a better getter, the better and better I do.

I work for Sam the silly simp
who slices slice sticks of slippery slimy sloppy salami;
at Snider's Salt Saccharin and seed store,
as I mashes, mentally and morally,
all musky musk Mellon in a matter of minutes,
at Carpenter's canned Catsup factory
in Canton Connecticut Continental United State. Rapp

How much wood could a wood chuck chuck
if a wood chuck could chuck wood?

Peter Piper picked a peck of pickled peppers.
A peck of pickled peppers Peter Piper picked.
When Peter Piper picked a peck of pickled peppers
a peck of pickled peppers Peter piper picked.

As I was walking up the stair,
I met a man who wasn't there.
He wasn't there again to day.
I wish I wish he'd go away. H. Mearns.

As I was sitting in my chair.
I knew the bottom wasn't there.
Nor back, nor side, but I just sat,
ignoring little things like that. H. Mearns.

Does your shirt shop stock short socks with spots?

Round and round the rugged rock the ragged rascal ran.

Of all the saws I ever saw, I never saw a saw saw like that saw saws.

Sixty six sick chicks.

The sun shines on the shop signs.

Six thick thistle sticks.

The sixth shiek's sixth sheep's sick.

Double bubble gum bubbles double trouble.

Rubber baby buggy bumpers. (Repeat three times.)

Eat fish fried fish free at the fish fry.

"Go my son and shut the shutter" This I heard a mother utter.
"Shutter's shut", the boy did mutter. "I can't shut'er any shutter."

Two tooters who tooted a flute
tried to tutor two tooters to toot.
"Is it harder to toot", said the two to the tutors,
"or to tutor two tutors to toot?

Cross crossing cautiously.

Supersonic, idiotic, disconnected, brain affected,
scubby dubby, dumb dumb.

Lemon liniment.

Tongue twisters twist tongues twisted trying to untangle twisted tangles.

UP TIGHT

Don Rapp Ph.D.

Nose to the grind stone,
shoulder to the wheel.
You're about as warm
as a cold blooded eel.

You work too hard.
You play too little.
You're exceedingly dull.
You're fat in the middle.

A type "A" personality;
tense all the time.
You're double up tight.
Your back's a straight line.

Death is tomorrow.
No more than next week,
unless you relax,
a-fish'in in the creek.

What more can I say.
I want you around.
I want you next week,
fit, healthy and sound.

You're very important.
You are a joy.
So take care of yourself;
you're much more than a toy.

THE CHANGING ME

Don Rapp

Once more I am . . .
different than before.
I'm altered to my very core.

I feel changed. But I'm ok.
I'm modified almost every day.

A mid life crisis? No no really not.
I'm just revamping what I've already got.

I was good, and now I'm better.
I'm friskier than an Irish Setter.

I'm thankful for all these events;
and much more hopeful, and a lot less tense;
about my future and my ability to do,
those things I aughta, and those things brand new.

Change is usual. Change is right.
Change increases my personal insight.

I'm not talking about perfection.
I'm talking about personal correction.

Tiny tiny changes that let me know
that life's never stiff, I'm still on the go.

Change is life, and life's great range,
is fostered better by my willingness to change.

Bibliography

Adams, C.C. *The Knot Book: An Elementary Introduction to the Mathematical Theory of Knots,* W.H. Freeman and Co., New York, NY. 1994

Armstrong, T. *Seven Kinds of Smart: Identifying and Developing Your Many Intelligences,* A Plume Book, Penguin Book, New York, NY. 1993

Beek, P J. and Lewbel, A., *The Science of Juggling: Studying the Ability to Toss and Catch Balls and Rings Provides Insight into Human Coordination, Robotics and Mathematics.* Scientific American, November. 1995

Benson, H. *Relaxation Response,* Avon. New York, NY. 1976

Booth F. et al. *Waging War on Modern Chronic Diseases: Primary Prevention through Exercise Biology.* In the American Psychological Society Report. 2001

Bortz, W. MD. *Dare to be 100.* A Fireside Book, Simon and Schuster, New York, NY, 1996

Bovre, S. *Balance Training: A Program for Improving Balance in Older Adults.* Desert Southwest Fitness, Tucson, AR. 2001

Bryson, L. Ed. *An Outline of Man's Knowledge of the Modern World.* Nelson Doubleday Inc. Garden City, NY, 1960

Burnette, J. Ed. American College of Sport Medicine, Exercise Leader Certification Class Materials. Christian Life Center. Tallahassee, Fl. 1997

Buzon, T. *Make the Most of Your Mind.* Linden Press, Simon and Schuster. New York, NY. 1984

Capacchione, L. *The Power of the Other Hand.* New Castle Pub Co. North Hollywood, CA, 1988

Chapman, E. *Attitude: Your Most Priceless Possession.* Crisp Pub Inc. Menlo Park, CA. 1990

Chapman, E. *Life is an Attitude: Staying Positive During Tough Times.* Crisp Pub Inc. Menlo Park, CA. 1992

Clark, K N. *Balance and Strength Training for Obese Individuals.* American College of Sports Medicine Health and Fitness Journal. January/February, Vol. 8/No. 2004

Colley, A.M. Beech, J.R. Editors. *Cognition and Action in Skilled Behavior.* Advance in Psychology 55. North-Holland. Amsterdam. 1988

Diamond, M. *Magic Trees of the Mind: How to Nurture Your Child's Intelligence, Creativity and Healthy Emotions from Birth Through Adolescence.* Dutton, Penguin Press. New York. NY. 1998

Engleman, M. *Aerobics of the Mind: Keeping the Mind Active in Aging. A New Perspective on Programming for Older Adults.* Venture Pub, Inc. State College, PA. 1996

Feldenkrais, M. *Awareness Through Movement: Health Exercises for Personal Growth.* Harper. San Francisco. CA. 1977. Paper Back 1990

Gardner, H. *Intelligence Reframed: Multiple Intelligences for the 21st Century.* Basic Book. New York, NY. 1999

Geithner, C. etal. *Personal Balance: Its Importance and How to Achieve It.* American College of Sports Medicine Health and fitness Journal. January/February. 2007

Gelb M, How *to Think Like Leonardo da Vinci: Seven Steps to Genius Every Day.* Delacorte Press. New York, NY. 1998

Gelb, J, and Buzon, T, *Lessons From the Art of Juggling.* Crown Trade Paperbacks, New York. NY. 1994

Gottlieb, R. *Attention and Memory Training for Children.* Based on the work of Dr. Robert Pepper, O.D. Lake Oswego OR, Self Published, No date given

Hannaford, C. *Smart Moves: Why Learning is not all in Your Head.* Great Ocean Pub. Arlington, VA. 1995

Hart, L. *How the Brain Works.* Basic Books. New York, NY. 1975

Hawkins, B A. May, M. Rogers, B. N. *Therapeutic Activity Intervention With The Elderly: Foundations and Practices.* Venture Pub, Inc. State College Pennsylvania, PA. 1996

Hooper, J. and Teresi, D. *The 3-Pound Universe: The Brain From the Chemistry of the Mind to the New Frontiers of the Soul.* Del Pub. Co. New York, NY. 1987

Horak, F. and Wolllacott, M. *Balance Disorders and Falls in the Elderly: A Course for Physical Therapist.* Orlando, Fl. September 1998

Jacobson, G. P. et al. *Handbook for Balance Function Testing.* Chapters, 7, 12, 13, 14, 15. 21, 22. Mosby Year Book. St Louis, MO. 1997

James W. *Psychology: The Briefer Course.* Dover Pub. Inc. Mineola, New York, NY. 2001. Originally published 1892

Johnson, A. *String Games: A Book of String Figures.* Klutz, Palo Alto, CA. 1993
Johnson, *A. Cat's Cradle: String Games from Around the World.* Klutz, Palo, Alto, CA. 1995

Jones J. and Rose D, Co-Editors, *Journal of Aging and Physical Activity.* Human Kinetics Pub. Champaign, IL 2005. Research Reference to the Aging and Physical Activity.

Journal of Creative Behavior. Pub. The Creative Education Foundation Inc. General Personal reading from 1990 – 2001

Kalb, C. *The Meaning of Falling.* Newsweek. Page 63, December. 11. 2000

Klaus H. et al. *Exercise Training for Rehabilitation and Secondary Prevention of Falls in Geriatric Patients with a History of Injurious Falls.* Journal of American Geriatrics Society. 49: 10 – 20. 2001

Kotulak, R. *Unlocking the Mind.* Chicago Tribune. Sunday, April 11. 1993

Kotulak, R, *Learning How to Use the Brain,* p 39, plus more good material on the brain. In Brain Development Research. Complied by: United Way of Florida. Statewide Success by 6 Workshop. Tampa, FL Sept 12 & 13 1996.

Masdeu, J. C, Ed. *Gait Disorders of Aging: Falls and Therapeutic Strategies.* Lippincott-Raven. 1997

Messer, M. *It's Ok to Play.* Writer's Digest. Page 22, July. 2001

Montagu, A. *Don't Be Adultish!* Psychology Today Magazine. P. 37. October, 1977

Montagu, A. *Growing Young.* McGraw-Hill Book Cooper. New York, NY, 1883

Nuland, S. *How We Live: The Brain and Human Nature. Mining the Mind,* Chaper 12, Vintage Books, Random House Inc. New York, NY. 1997

Peale, N.V. *The Power of Positive Thinking.* Prentice-Hall. Englewood Cliffs, NJ. 1978

Perkins-Carpenters, B. *How to Prevent Falls: A Comprehensive Guide to Better Balance.* Senior Fitness Production, Inc. New York, NY. 1999

Perry B. D. MD. *Incubated in Terror: Neurodevelpmental Factors in the Cycle of Violence.* P 87. Plus more good material on the brain. In Brain Development Research. Complied by: United Way of Florida. Statewide Success by 6 Workshop. Tampa, FL Sept 12 & 13, 1996.

Perry, G. Knots. A Practical step-by-step Guide to Tying over 100 Knots. Barnes and Noble. New York, NY. 2002

Rapp, D. *Become Your Own Balance Coach.* Class manual Self Pub. Tallahassee, FL. 1999

Ratey, John J. *A User User's Guide to the Brain. Perception, Attention, and the Four Theaters of the Brain.* Pantheon Book. New York, NY 2001

Rediger, G. L, *Fit To Be A Pastor: A Call to Physical, Mental, and Spiritual Fitness.* Westminster John Knox Press, Louisville, KY. 2000

Reichler, G. *Active Wellness: A Personalized 10 Step Program for a Healthy Body, Mind and Spirit.* Time Warner Books. 1998

Restak, R. *Mozart's Brain and the Fighter Pilot: Unleashing Your Brain's Potential.* Harmony Books, Random House. New York, NY. 2001

Rikli, R. and Jones J. *Senior Fitness Test Manual.* Human Kinetics. Champaign, IL 2000

Rose, D. Fall Proof. Human Kinetics. Champaign, IL 2003

Rouillard, L. A. *Goals and Goal Setting: Planning to Succeed.* Crisp Pub Inc. Menlo Park, CA. 1993

Spirduso, W. *Physical Dimension of Aging.* Human Kinetics. Champaign, IL. 1995

Steinberg, M & Othmer, S. *ADD: The 200 Hour Solution: Training Minds to Concentrate and Self-Regulate Naturally Without Medication.* Robert D. Reed Pub, Bandon, OR. 2004

Sunbeck, D. *Infinity Walk: The Physical Self.* Leonardo Foundation Press. 2002

Travell, J. & Simons. L *Myofascial Pain and Dysfunction: The Trigger Point Manual.* Second Ed. Vol. 1 & 2. Lippincott Williams & Wilkins, USA. 1999

Weinstein M. and Goodman. J. *Playfair: Everybody's Guide to Noncompetitive Play.* Impact Pub. San Luis Obispo, CA. 1980

Woollacott. *A: The manipulation of Sensory Input of the Somatosensory, Visual, Vestibular and Systems.* Journal of Gerontology, 49, 52 - 71. 1994

Zorpette. Glenn. *Muscular Again.* Scientific American, November, 1999

Index

ON BALANCE: MASTERY OF PHYSICAL BALANCE FOR LIFE

The message is clear.
Balance can be enhanced.

You or a family member or friend may have need for better balance. Please know that more secure, life-long balance is possible. On Balance offers many suggestions that can be used to better your daily life.

On Balance chapters include:

- **Fitness**
- **Motivation**
- **The brain's responsibility for balance**
- **Neurological systems that control balance**
- **Knowledge tools to manage balance**
- **Physical tools to keep the nervous system alert**
- **Bibliography, appendix and index**

Contact - Don Rapp:
Email - Rappdp@aol.com

Phone - 850-385-5627

Book - $20.00 Shipping & Handling - $3.00 Total $23.00
Check only - payable to - Don Rapp

Don Rapp, 4156 Covenant Lane, Tallahassee, FL 32308

The Web site contains information and suggestions to prevent falls, Solid, upright balance is the goal.